The American Psychiatric Association Practice Guideline for the Treatment of Patients With Borderline Personality Disorder

SECOND EDITION

Guideline Writing Group
George A. Keepers, M.D. (Chair)
Laura J. Fochtmann, M.D., M.B.I. (Vice-Chair; Methodologist)
Joan M. Anzia, M.D.
Sheldon Benjamin, M.D.
Jeffrey M. Lyness, M.D.
Ramin Mojtabai, M.D.
Mark Servis, M.D.
Lois Choi-Kain, M.D.
Kaz J. Nelson, M.D.
John M. Oldham, M.D.
Carla Sharp, Ph.D.
Amanda Degenhardt, M.D.

Systematic Review Group
Laura J. Fochtmann, M.D., M.B.I. (Methodologist)
John M. Oldham, M.D.
Seung-Hee Hong

Committee on Practice Guidelines
Daniel J. Anzia, M.D. (Chair)
R. Scott Benson, M.D.
Oscar G. Bukstein, M.D.
Catherine Crone, M.D.
Jacqueline Posada, M.D.
Michael J. Vergare, M.D.
Ilse Wiechers, M.D.
Muniza Majoka, M.D. (Corresponding Member)
Saundra Stock, M.D. (Corresponding Member)
Rochelle Woods, M.D. (Corresponding Member)
Joel Yager, M.D. (Corresponding Member)
Laura J. Fochtmann, M.D., M.B.I. (Consultant)

APA Assembly Liaisons
Daniel Dahl, M.D.
Evan Eyler, M.D.
Harold Ginsburg, M.D.
Jason W. Hunziker, M.D.
Marvin Koss, M.D.
Lisa Schock, M.D.
Ilse Wiechers, M.D.
Brian Zimnitsky, M.D.

APA and the Guideline Writing Group especially thank Laura J. Fochtmann, M.D., M.B.I., Seung-Hee Hong, and Jennifer Medicus for their outstanding work and effort in developing this guideline. APA also wishes to acknowledge the contributions of other APA staff including Kristin Kroeger Ptakowski. APA wishes to give special recognition to John M. Oldham, M.D., for his decades of contributions to APA and its practice guidelines, including his work on the current guideline as part of the Systematic Review and Guideline Writing Groups and serving as Chair of the writing group for the prior version of this guideline. APA also thanks the APA Committee on Practice Guidelines (Daniel J. Anzia, M.D., Chair), liaisons from the APA Assembly for their input and assistance, and APA Councils and others for providing feedback during the comment period.

For inquiries about permissions or licensing, please contact Permissions & Licensing, American Psychiatric Association Publishing, 800 Maine Avenue SW, Suite 900, Washington, DC 20024-2812 or submit inquiries online at: www.appi.org/Support/Customer-Information/Permissions.

If you wish to buy 50 or more copies of the same title, please go to www.appi.org/specialdiscounts for more information.

Second Edition

Manufactured in the United States of America on acid-free paper
27 26 25 24   5 4 3 2

American Psychiatric Association
800 Maine Avenue SW, Suite 900
Washington, DC 20024-2812
www.appi.org

Library of Congress Cataloging-in-Publication Data

Names: American Psychiatric Association, author, publisher. | American Psychiatric Association. Work Group on Borderline Personality Disorder. Practice guideline for the treatment of patients with borderline personality disorder.
Title: The American Psychiatric Association practice guideline for the treatment of patients with borderline personality disorder.
Other titles: Practice guideline for the treatment of patients with borderline personality disorder
Description: Second edition. | Washington, DC : American Psychiatric Association, [2025] | Preceded by Practice guideline for the treatment of patients with borderline personality disorder / [Work Group on Borderline Personality Disorder]. c2001. | Includes bibliographical references.
Identifiers: LCCN 2024020490 (print) | LCCN 2024020491 (ebook) | ISBN 9780890427095 (paperback) | ISBN 9780890427101 (ebook)
Subjects: MESH: Borderline Personality Disorder--therapy | Psychotherapy--methods | Practice Guideline
Classification: LCC RC569.5.B67 (print) | LCC RC569.5.B67 (ebook) | NLM WM 190.5.B5 | DDC 616.85/85206--dc23/eng/20240603
LC record available at https://lccn.loc.gov/2024020490
LC ebook record available at https://lccn.loc.gov/2024020491

British Library Cataloguing in Publication Data
A CIP record is available from the British Library.

Contents

Acronyms/Abbreviations v

Introduction 1

    Rationale 1

    Scope of Document 3

        Scope Constraints Related to the Systematic
        Review of Evidence 3

        Scope Constraints Related to the Alternative DSM-5 Model for
        Personality Disorders 4

    Overview of the Development Process 4

    Rating the Strengths of Guideline Statements and Supporting
    Research Evidence 5

    Proper Use of Guidelines 6

Guideline Statement Summary 7

    Assessment and Determination of Treatment Plan 7

    Psychosocial Interventions 7

    Pharmacotherapy. 7

Guideline Statements and Implementation 9

    Assessment and Determination of Treatment Plan 9

    Statement 1 – Initial Assessment 9

        Implementation. 9

    Statement 2 – Quantitative Measures. 15

        Implementation. 15

    Statement 3 – Treatment Planning 18

        Implementation 18

    Statement 4 – Discussion of Diagnosis and Treatment 32

        Implementation 32

Psychosocial Interventions. 33

    Statement 5 – Psychotherapy 33

        Implementation 33

    Pharmacotherapy 37

    Statement 6 – Clinical Review Before Medication Initiation 37

        Implementation 37

    Statement 7 – Pharmacotherapy Principles 38

        Implementation 38

    Statement 8 – Pharmacotherapy Review 39

        Implementation 39

Areas for Further Research 41

    Methodological Issues 41

    Research Topics. 42

    Prevention, Screening, and Assessment. 42

    Treatment Planning 43

    Ethical Issues in BPD Assessment and Treatment 44

Guideline Development Process 47

    Management of Potential Conflicts of Interest. 47

    Guideline Writing Group Composition 47

    Systematic Review Methodology. 47

    Rating the Strength of Supporting Research Evidence 48

    Rating the Strength of Guideline Statements. 49

    Use of Guidelines to Enhance Quality of Care. 50

    External Review 51

    Funding and Approval 52

References. 53

Disclosures 79

Individuals and Organizations That Submitted Comments 83

Acronyms/Abbreviations

ADHD=attention-deficit/hyperactivity disorder

AHRQ=Agency for Healthcare Research and Quality

AMPD=alternative model for personality disorders

APA=American Psychiatric Association

ASD=autism spectrum disorder

AUD=alcohol use disorder

BEST=Borderline Evaluation of Severity Over Time

BPD=borderline personality disorder

BSL-23=Borderline Symptom List 23-item

CBT=cognitive-behavioral therapy

DBT=dialectical behavior therapy

DDP=dynamic deconstructive psychotherapy

DERS=Difficulty in Emotional Regulation Scale

DSHI=Deliberate Self-Harm Inventory

DSM=*Diagnostic and Statistical Manual of Mental Disorders*

DSM-5-TR=*Diagnostic and Statistical Manual of Mental Disorders*, 5th Edition, Text Revision

ECT=electroconvulsive therapy

EMDR=eye movement desensitization and reprocessing

GPM=good psychiatric management

GRADE=Grading of Recommendations Assessment, Development and Evaluation

HIPAA=Health Insurance Portability and Accountability Act

ICD-10=*International Statistical Classification of Diseases and Related Health Problems*, 10th Revision

LAI=long-acting injectable

LPFS-BF=Level of Personality Functioning Scale–Brief Form 2.0

MAOI=monoamine oxidase inhibitor

MBT=mentalization-based treatment

MDD=major depressive disorder

MDMA=3, 4-methylenedioxymethamphetamine

NSSI=non-suicidal self-injury

OCD=obsessive-compulsive disorder

PROMIS=Patient-Reported Outcomes Measurement Information System

PTSD=posttraumatic stress disorder

RCT=randomized controlled trial

SFT=schema-focused therapy

SOFAS=Social and Occupational Functioning Assessment Scale

SSRI=selective serotonin reuptake inhibitor

STEPPS=Systems Training for Emotional Predictability and Problem Solving

SUD=substance use disorder

TFP=transference-focused psychotherapy

TMS=transcranial magnetic stimulation

WHODAS 2.0=World Health Organization Disability Schedule 2.0

ZAN-BPD=Zanarini Rating Scale for Borderline Personality Disorder

Introduction

Rationale

The goal of this guideline is to improve the quality of care and treatment outcomes for patients with borderline personality disorder (BPD) as defined in Section II of the *Diagnostic and Statistical Manual of Mental Disorders*, 5th Edition, Text Revision (DSM-5-TR; American Psychiatric Association 2022a). Since publication of the last American Psychiatric Association (APA) practice guideline (American Psychiatric Association 2001) and guideline watch on BPD (Oldham 2005), there have been many studies on psychotherapies for individuals with BPD as well as some studies on pharmacotherapies. Despite this, there are still misconceptions about BPD (Baker and Beazley 2022; Masland et al. 2023; Proctor et al. 2021; Sheehan et al. 2016; Stiles et al. 2023) and substantial gaps in the availability of evidence-based treatments for individuals with BPD (Iliakis et al. 2019; Lohman et al. 2017). This practice guideline aims to help clinicians improve the care and well-being of their patients by reviewing current evidence and providing evidence-based statements intended to enhance knowledge and optimize treatment of BPD.

BPD is characterized in DSM-5-TR as being associated with a long-term pattern of instability of interpersonal relationships, unstable self-image, marked impulsivity, and/or affective instability (American Psychiatric Association 2022a). In addition, these features can be evidenced by efforts to avoid real or feared abandonment, chronic feelings of emptiness, mood reactivity, recurrent self-injurious or suicidal behavior, other impulsive behaviors with potential for self-damaging effects, intense anger or difficulty with anger control, and transient paranoid ideation or stress-related dissociative symptoms (American Psychiatric Association 2022a).

As with personality disorders in general, the pattern of inner experience and behavior with BPD can be quite heterogeneous but is relatively pervasive and enduring (American Psychiatric Association 2022a). Symptom onset may extend back to early adolescence, although the diagnosis of BPD may not be made until later in adolescence or adulthood (American Psychiatric Association 2022a). In addition, it occurs across a broad range of personal and social situations, is markedly different from the expectations of the individual's cultural or societal norms, and leads to clinically significant distress or impairment in social, occupational, or other important areas of functioning (American Psychiatric Association 2022a). Although co-occurring conditions are common, the specific features of the personality disorder are not better explained by the effects of a substance, another psychiatric disorder, or another medical disorder (American Psychiatric Association 2022a).

The lifetime prevalence of BPD in the United States is approximately 1.4%–2.7%, although estimates can vary depending on the study location, sample demographic characteristics, and case finding and diagnostic approaches (Ellison et al. 2018; Grant et al. 2008; Leichsenring et al. 2023; Lenzenweger et al. 2007; Trull et al. 2010; Volkert et al. 2018; Winsper et al. 2020). In clinical populations, women are more frequently diagnosed with BPD and tend to seek treatment more often than men; however, nonclinical samples suggest that the prevalence of BPD is likely to be comparable in men and women (Busch et al. 2016; Lenzenweger et al. 2007; Zanarini et al. 2011a). Few studies have assessed the prevalence of BPD in LGBTQ+ individuals (Denning et al. 2022; Rodriguez-Seijas et al. 2021). An estimated three-quarters of patients with BPD seek help from professional mental health services (Tomko et al. 2014). In clinical psychiatric populations, the prevalence of BPD is high and estimated at 10%–18% for outpatients and 9%–25% for inpatients (Doering 2019;

Ellison et al. 2018; Gunderson 2009; Torgersen 2005; Volkert et al. 2018; Zimmerman et al. 2017). Individuals with BPD are also frequent users of primary care (Doering 2019) and have elevated rates of chronic pain and other somatic conditions (El-Gabalawy et al. 2010; Heath et al. 2018b; Sansone and Sansone 2012; Tate et al. 2022). The lifetime prevalence of BPD among primary care patients is about four times as high as in the general population (Gross et al. 2002). A high prevalence of BPD (21%) was also found among veterans receiving care in U.S. Veterans Health Centers (Edwards et al. 2022).

Individuals with BPD commonly have other psychiatric disorders such as major depressive disorder (MDD), bipolar disorder, posttraumatic stress disorder (PTSD), anxiety disorders, eating disorders, attention-deficit/hyperactivity disorder (ADHD), substance use disorders (SUDs), and other personality disorders (Choi-Kain et al. 2022; Friborg et al. 2014; Geluk Rouwhorst et al. 2023; Grant et al. 2016; Gunderson et al. 2014; Keuroghlian et al. 2015; Leichsenring et al. 2011; Lenzenweger et al. 2007; McDermid et al. 2015; McGlashan et al. 2000; Miller et al. 2022; Momen et al. 2022; Philipsen et al. 2008; Santo et al. 2022; Tate et al. 2022; Trull et al. 2018; Zanarini et al. 2004a, 2010, 2019; Zimmerman et al. 2017). Most individuals with BPD will usually present first for treatment of another disorder, such as a mood or anxiety disorder (Zimmerman et al. 2017). Furthermore, when a co-occurring disorder is present, the clinical presentation may be more severe, and symptom remission is often more difficult to achieve in the co-occurring disorder (Ceresa et al. 2021; Geluk Rouwhorst et al. 2023; Gunderson et al. 2014; Keuroghlian et al. 2015; Skodol et al. 2011).

The lifetime burden and psychosocial impairment associated with BPD can be substantial because it typically has an onset in adolescence or early adulthood and can persist for many years (American Psychiatric Association 2022a; Doering 2019; Leichsenring et al. 2011; Oldham 2006). The lived experience of BPD can be associated with significant emotional pain and a diminished quality of life (Botter et al. 2021; Miller et al. 2021; Ng et al. 2019a, 2019b). Disruptions in relationships, including those with family, friends, and intimate partners, are common (Ng et al. 2019a, 2019b). Individuals with BPD may also experience disruptions in schooling, employment, and housing (Juurlink et al. 2019; Ng et al. 2019a, 2019b; Soloff 2021). Economic stability and productivity can be affected for those with BPD as well as for family members (Hastrup et al. 2019; Kay et al. 2018; Soloff 2021). In addition, individuals with BPD experience increases in health care costs related to BPD and to other physical conditions (Hastrup et al. 2019). These increases in costs can affect access to treatment and, in turn, affect health and quality of life (Lohman et al. 2017). Some studies suggest that individuals with BPD have an increased possibility of contacts with the criminal justice system (Dean et al. 2020; Nakic et al. 2022; Tate et al. 2022). Conversely, there are strong associations between having a diagnosis of BPD and being the victim of a violent crime (Tate et al. 2022). These significant consequences of BPD support a need for early identification and treatment.

In contrast to earlier views on BPD, this condition can remit, and symptoms can be reduced and managed. Most individuals with BPD will experience some decline in symptoms during adulthood (Gunderson et al. 2011; Stone 2017; Zanarini et al. 2012), and in clinical samples, about 85% of individuals with BPD will no longer meet the threshold for diagnosis within 10 years of longitudinal follow-up (Gunderson et al. 2011; Stone 2017; Zanarini et al. 2012). Nevertheless, specific symptoms such as fear of abandonment, impulsivity, intense anger, and an unstable self-image may persist. Individuals with BPD may also continue to experience impairments in social (Gunderson et al. 2011) and occupational functioning (Niesten et al. 2016) and may have a need for ongoing treatment.

Rates of suicide attempts and episodes of self-harm also decline over time (Zanarini et al. 2008), but they continue to occur more often than in individuals without BPD (Grilo and Udo 2021; Yen et al. 2021; Zanarini et al. 2008). Furthermore, in longitudinal studies, BPD is associated with increases in deaths due to suicide as well as with all-cause mortality (Kjær et al. 2020; Paris 2019; Schneider et al. 2019; Temes et al. 2019). Accordingly, an overall goal of this guideline is to enhance the assessment and treatment of BPD, thereby reducing the mortality, morbidity, and significant psychosocial and health consequences of this important psychiatric condition.

An additional rationale for this practice guideline is to provide clinicians with the necessary knowledge to feel confident in their skills for treating patients with BPD. A considerable amount of stigma exists in relation to BPD, including self-stigma, and patients with BPD often experience discrimination within the health care system (Baker and Beazley 2022; Masland et al. 2023; Proctor et al. 2021; Stiles et al. 2023). Bias about BPD is lessened and empathy for patients is increased when clinicians have received education about working with patients with this diagnosis (e.g., through seminars on good psychiatric management [GPM]; Keuroghlian et al. 2016; Klein et al. 2022b; Masland et al. 2018). It is also important for clinicians to gain perspectives on the lived experiences of these individuals. Other misconceptions about BPD can also be corrected through education. For example, one misconception is that BPD only occurs in adults; however, adolescents can meet criteria for the disorder and can benefit from treatment aimed at addressing its core features and symptoms (Bo et al. 2021; Ilagan and Choi-Kain 2021; Sharp 2017; Weiner et al. 2018; Winsper 2021). Education can also be helpful in emphasizing that treatment of BPD is effective and that many patients with BPD will improve with treatment (Bohus et al. 2021; Gunderson et al. 2011; Leichsenring et al. 2023; Stone 2017; Zanarini et al. 2012). Consequently, this guideline also aims to improve the quality of care for patients by providing clinicians with up-to-date knowledge about treating BPD.

Scope of Document

This practice guideline focuses on evidence-based treatments for BPD. In addition, it includes statements related to assessment and treatment planning, which are an integral part of patient-centered care.

Scope Constraints Related to the Systematic Review of Evidence

The scope of this document is shaped by recent diagnostic criteria for BPD as defined by DSM-IV, DSM-IV-TR, DSM-5, or ICD-10 and by the available evidence (American Psychiatric Association 1994, 2000, 2013a; World Health Organization 1992). The document scope is also affected by a number of limitations of the evidence as obtained by a systematic review of the literature through September 2021. Most studies enrolled predominantly White participants, but many studies did not specify the racial, ethnic, or cultural characteristics of the sample. Also, studies typically included a greater proportion of women than men. Furthermore, most studies reported the sex of participants but not their gender identity. Although we recognize the distinctions between sex and gender identity of participants, we have used the descriptions provided by the researchers, which may not align with currently accepted practice. Our review included research with participants ages 13 and older, and some studies were focused specifically on adolescents. Other studies primarily included adult populations or did not analyze data based on age. Furthermore, key issues of relevance to adolescents and emerging adults such as family relationships and trajectories of psychosocial development were not systematically assessed. These gaps emphasize the compelling need for additional research in more representative samples.

The lived experience of individuals with BPD is another crucial topic where research has been sparse in terms both of BPD symptoms and their impact and of treatment-related experiences and how they may influence treatment outcomes.

Data are also limited on the treatment of individuals with BPD who also have significant physical health conditions or co-occurring psychiatric conditions, including SUDs. Many of the available studies of BPD did not analyze data separately for these patient subgroups or excluded individuals with these comorbidities. Few studies were specifically aimed at examining effectiveness of treatment in individuals with BPD and a co-occurring condition. Nevertheless, in the absence of more robust evidence, the statements in this guideline should generally be applicable to individuals with co-occurring conditions.

Our systematic review did not include studies related to risk factors of BPD, prevention of BPD, complex PTSD, or non-suicidal self-injury (NSSI) in the absence of other BPD features. It also did not include search terms to identify literature on stigma and discrimination, either as risk factors for BPD, contributors to morbidity, or barriers to seeking treatment. Each of these topics is important but would warrant a distinct systematic review from one focused on treatments for BPD.

Cost-effectiveness considerations and the availability of specific treatments are also outside of the scope of this guideline. Although availability and cost are often barriers to receiving treatment, each of these factors typically differs by country and geographical region and varies widely with the health system and payment model. In addition, few high-quality studies exist on the cost-effectiveness of treatments for BPD that could be utilized to inform health care policy.

Finally, we do not discuss telehealth as a specific intervention because no studies with direct comparisons of telehealth and in-person care met the inclusion criteria for the systematic review. Research on the use of telehealth, Web-based interventions, and mobile applications is rapidly expanding, however, which will help to inform future practice guidelines.

Scope Constraints Related to the Alternative DSM-5 Model for Personality Disorders

We recognize that the Alternative DSM-5 Model for Personality Disorders (AMPD; DSM-5-TR, Section III: "Emerging Measures and Models," American Psychiatric Association 2022a) has had a significant impact in the realm of personality disorder assessment (Krueger and Hobbs 2020; Zimmermann et al. 2019) and is useful in adolescents as well as adults (Sharp et al. 2022). The AMPD is increasingly being integrated into clinical practice (Bach and Tracy 2022; Milinkovic and Tiliopoulos 2020; Oldham 2022a). From both diagnostic and treatment standpoints, it is helpful to determine whether core impairments are present in self-functioning (i.e., identity and self-direction) and in interpersonal functioning (i.e., empathy and intimacy) (American Psychiatric Association 2022a; Sharp and Wall 2021). Despite the growing recognition of the importance of the AMPD, our systematic review did not identify treatment studies using the AMPD that met our inclusion criteria. Thus, we are including it as an area that requires further treatment-related research, but we have not incorporated it into our recommendations in this version of the practice guideline.

Overview of the Development Process

Since the publication of the Institute of Medicine (now known as the National Academy of Medicine) report *Clinical Practice Guidelines We Can Trust* (Institute of Medicine 2011), there has been an increasing focus on using clearly defined, transparent processes for rating the quality of evidence and the strength of the overall body of evidence in systematic reviews of the scientific literature. This guideline was developed using a process intended to be consistent with the recommendations of the Institute of Medicine (2011) and the "Principles for the Development of Specialty Society Clinical Guidelines" of the Council of Medical Specialty Societies (2017). Parameters used for the guideline's systematic review are included with the full text and the appendices of the guideline; the development process is fully described in the following document available on the APA Web site: www.psychiatry.org/psychiatrists/practice/clinical-practice-guidelines/guideline-development-process

Rating the Strengths of Guideline Statements and Supporting Research Evidence

Development of guideline statements entails weighing the potential benefits and harms of the statement and then identifying the level of confidence in that determination. This concept of balancing benefits and harms to determine guideline recommendations and strength of recommendations is a hallmark of GRADE (Grading of Recommendations Assessment, Development and Evaluation), which is used by many professional organizations around the world to develop practice guideline recommendations (Guyatt et al. 2013). With the GRADE approach, recommendations are rated by assessing the confidence that the benefits of the statement outweigh its harms and burdens, determining the confidence in estimates of effect as reflected by the quality of evidence, estimating patient values and preferences (including whether they are similar across the patient population), and identifying whether resource expenditures are worth the expected net benefit of following the recommendation (Andrews et al. 2013).

In weighing the balance of benefits and harms for each statement in this guideline, our level of confidence is informed by available evidence, which includes evidence from clinical trials as well as expert opinion and patient values and preferences. Evidence for the benefit of a particular intervention within a specific clinical context is identified through systematic review and is then balanced against the evidence for harms. In this regard, *harms* are broadly defined and may include serious adverse events, less serious adverse events that affect tolerability, minor adverse events, negative effects of the intervention on quality of life, barriers and inconveniences associated with treatment, direct and indirect costs of the intervention (including opportunity costs), and other negative aspects of the treatment that may influence decision making by the patient, the clinician, or both.

Many topics covered in this guideline have relied on forms of evidence such as consensus opinions of experienced clinicians or indirect findings from observational studies rather than research from randomized trials. It is well recognized that there are guideline topics and clinical circumstances for which high-quality evidence from clinical trials is not possible or is unethical to obtain (Council of Medical Specialty Societies 2017). For example, many questions need to be asked as part of an assessment, and inquiring about a particular symptom or element of the history cannot be separated out for study as a discrete intervention. It would also be impossible to separate changes in outcomes due to assessment from changes in outcomes due to ensuing treatment. Research on psychiatric assessments and some psychiatric interventions can also be complicated by multiple confounding factors such as the interaction between the clinician and the patient or the patient's unique circumstances and experiences. The GRADE working group and guidelines developed by other professional organizations have noted that a strong recommendation or "good practice statement" may be appropriate even in the absence of research evidence when sensible alternatives do not exist (Andrews et al. 2013; Brito et al. 2013; Djulbegovic et al. 2009; Hazlehurst et al. 2013). For each guideline statement, we have described the type and strength of the available evidence as well as the factors, including patient preferences, that were used in determining the balance of benefits and harms.

The authors of the guideline determined each final rating, as described in the section "Guideline Development Process" (see Table 1). A *recommendation* (denoted by the numeral 1 after the guideline statement) indicates confidence that the benefits of the intervention clearly outweigh the harms. A *suggestion* (denoted by the numeral 2 after the guideline statement) indicates greater uncertainty. Although the benefits of the statement are still viewed as outweighing the harms, the balance of benefits and harms is more difficult to judge, or either the benefits or the harms may be less clear. With a suggestion, patient values and preferences may be more variable, and this can influence the clinical decision that is ultimately made. Each guideline statement also has an associated

TABLE 1. Rating the strengths of guideline statements and evidence for guideline statements

Strength of guideline statement			Strength of evidence		
1	Recommendation	Denotes confidence that the benefits of the intervention clearly outweigh the harms.	A	High confidence	Further research is very unlikely to change the estimate of effect and our confidence in it.
2	Suggestion	Denotes benefits that are viewed as outweighing harms, but the balance is more difficult to judge and patient values and preferences may be more variable.	B	Moderate confidence	Further research may change the estimate of effect and our confidence in it.
			C	Low confidence	Further research is likely to change the estimate of effect and our confidence in it.

rating for the *strength of supporting research evidence*. Three ratings are used: *high, moderate,* and *low* (denoted by the letters A, B, and C, respectively) and reflect the level of confidence that the evidence for a guideline statement reflects a true effect based on consistency of findings across studies, directness of the effect on a specific health outcome, precision of the estimate of effect, and risk of bias in available studies (Agency for Healthcare Research and Quality 2014; Balshem et al. 2011; Guyatt et al. 2006).

Proper Use of Guidelines

APA Practice Guidelines are assessments of current (as of the date of authorship) scientific and clinical information provided as an educational service. The guidelines 1) do not set a standard of care and are not inclusive of all proper treatments or methods of care; 2) are not continually updated and may not reflect the most recent evidence, as new evidence may emerge between the time information is developed and when the guidelines are published or read; 3) address only the question(s) or issue(s) specifically identified; 4) do not mandate any particular course of medical care; 5) are not intended to substitute for the independent professional judgment of the treating clinician; and 6) do not account for individual variation among patients. As such, it is not possible to draw conclusions about the effects of omitting a particular recommendation, either in general or for a specific patient. Furthermore, adherence to these guidelines will not ensure a successful outcome for every individual, nor should these guidelines be interpreted as including all proper methods of evaluation and care or excluding other acceptable methods of evaluation and care aimed at the same results. The ultimate recommendation regarding a particular assessment, clinical procedure, or treatment plan must be made by the clinician directly involved in the patient's care in light of the psychiatric evaluation, other clinical data, and the diagnostic and treatment options available. Such recommendations should be made in collaboration with the patient whenever possible and should incorporate the patient's personal and sociocultural preferences and values in order to enhance the therapeutic alliance, adherence to treatment, and treatment outcomes. For all these reasons, the APA cautions against the use of guidelines in litigation. Use of these guidelines is voluntary. APA provides the guidelines on an "as is" basis and makes no warranty, expressed or implied, regarding them. APA assumes no responsibility for any injury or damage to persons or property arising out of or related to any use of the guidelines or for any errors or omissions.

The appendixes for this guideline, including evidence tables, literature search results, clinical questions, and more, are available online at https://psychiatryonline.org/doi/book/10.1176/appi.books.9780890428009.

Guideline Statement Summary

Assessment and Determination of Treatment Plan

1. APA *recommends* **(1C)** that the initial assessment of a patient with possible borderline personality disorder include the reason the individual is presenting for evaluation; the patient's goals and preferences for treatment; a review of psychiatric symptoms, including core features of personality disorders and common co-occurring disorders; a psychiatric treatment history; an assessment of physical health; an assessment of psychosocial and cultural factors; a mental status examination; and an assessment of risk of suicide, self-injury, and aggressive behaviors, as outlined in APA's *Practice Guidelines for the Psychiatric Evaluation of Adults*, 3rd Edition.
2. APA *suggests* **(2C)** that the initial psychiatric evaluation of a patient with possible borderline personality disorder include a quantitative measure to identify and determine the severity of symptoms and impairments of functioning that may be a focus of treatment.
3. APA *recommends* **(1C)** that a patient with borderline personality disorder have a documented, comprehensive, and person-centered treatment plan.
4. APA *recommends* **(1C)** that a patient with borderline personality disorder be engaged in a collaborative discussion about their diagnosis and treatment, which includes psychoeducation related to the disorder.

Psychosocial Interventions

5. APA *recommends* **(1B)** that a patient with borderline personality disorder be treated with a structured approach to psychotherapy that has support in the literature and targets the core features of the disorder.

Pharmacotherapy

6. APA *recommends* **(1C)** that a patient with borderline personality disorder have a review of co-occurring disorders, prior psychotherapies, other nonpharmacological treatments, past medication trials, and current medications before initiating any new medication.
7. APA *suggests* **(2C)** that any psychotropic medication treatment of borderline personality disorder be time-limited, aimed at addressing a specific measurable target symptom, and adjunctive to psychotherapy.
8. APA *recommends* **(1C)** that a patient with borderline personality disorder receive a review and reconciliation of their medications at least every 6 months to assess the effectiveness of treatment and identify medications that warrant tapering or discontinuation.

Guideline Statements and Implementation

Assessment and Determination of Treatment Plan

Statement 1 – Initial Assessment

APA *recommends* **(1C)** that the initial assessment of a patient with possible borderline personality disorder include the reason the individual is presenting for evaluation; the patient's goals and preferences for treatment; a review of psychiatric symptoms, including core features of personality disorders and common co-occurring disorders; a psychiatric treatment history; an assessment of physical health; an assessment of psychosocial and cultural factors; a mental status examination; and an assessment of risk of suicide, self-injury, and aggressive behaviors, as outlined in APA's *Practice Guidelines for the Psychiatric Evaluation of Adults*, 3rd Edition.

Implementation

The importance of the psychiatric evaluation cannot be underestimated because it serves as the initial basis for a therapeutic relationship with the patient and provides information that is crucial to differential diagnosis and shared decision-making about treatment. The initial evaluation can also provide an opportunity for educating patients, family members, friends, or others involved in the patient's care about such factors as BPD features, treatments, course, and prognosis. APA's *Practice Guidelines for the Psychiatric Evaluation of Adults*, 3rd Edition (American Psychiatric Association 2016a), describes recommended and suggested elements of assessment for any individual who presents with psychiatric symptoms (Table 2). These elements are by no means comprehensive, and additional areas of inquiry will become apparent as the evaluation unfolds, depending on the responses to initial questions, the presenting concerns, the observations of the clinician during the assessment, the complexity and urgency of clinical decision-making, and other aspects of the clinical context. In many circumstances, aspects of the evaluation will extend across multiple visits (American Psychiatric Association 2016a).

The specific approach to the interview will depend on many factors, including the patient's ability to communicate, degree of cooperation, level of insight, illness severity, and ability to recall historical details (American Psychiatric Association 2016a). Such factors as the patient's health literacy (Clausen et al. 2016) and cultural background (Lewis-Fernández et al. 2016) can also influence their understanding or interpretation of questions. Typically, a psychiatric evaluation involves a direct interview between the patient and the clinician (American Psychiatric Association 2016a). The use of open-ended, empathic questions about the patient's current life circumstances and reasons for evaluation can provide an initial picture of the person and serve as a way of establishing rapport. Such questions can be followed up with additional structured inquiry about history, symptoms, or observations made during the assessment.

A respectful and empathic approach to the interview is important because patients may have had prior experiences with stigma or bias in health care settings or may have self-stigmatizing views (Denning et al. 2022; Goldhammer et al. 2019; Klein et al. 2022a; Masland et al. 2023; McKenzie et al. 2022; Olbert et al. 2018; Rodriguez-Seijas et al. 2023; Schwartz and Blankenship 2014; Stiles

TABLE 2. **Recommended aspects of the initial psychiatric evaluation**

History of present illness

Reason the patient is presenting for evaluation, including current symptoms, behaviors, and precipitating factors

Current psychiatric diagnoses and psychiatric review of systems

Psychiatric history

Hospitalization and emergency department visits for psychiatric issues, including substance use disorders

Psychiatric treatments (type, duration, and, where applicable, doses)

Response and adherence to psychiatric treatments, including psychosocial treatments, pharmacotherapy, and other interventions such as electroconvulsive therapy or transcranial magnetic stimulation

Prior psychiatric diagnoses and symptoms, including

- Hallucinations (including command hallucinations), delusions, and negative symptoms
- Aggressive ideas or behaviors (e.g., homicide, domestic or workplace violence, other physically or sexually aggressive threats or acts)
- Impulsivity
- Suicidal ideas, suicide plans, and suicide attempts, including details of each attempt (e.g., context, method, damage, potential lethality, intent) and attempts that were aborted or interrupted
- Intentional self-injury in which there was no suicide intent

Substance use history

Use of tobacco, alcohol, and other substances (e.g., vaping, marijuana, cocaine, heroin, hallucinogens) and any misuse of prescribed or over-the-counter medications or supplements

Current or recent substance use disorder or change in use of alcohol or other substances

Medical history

Whether or not the patient has an ongoing relationship with a primary care health professional

Allergies or drug sensitivities

All medications patient is currently taking or has recently taken and side effects of these medications (i.e., both prescribed and nonprescribed medications, herbal and nutritional supplements, and vitamins)

Past or current medical illnesses and related hospitalizations

Relevant past or current treatments, including surgeries, other procedures, or complementary and alternative medical treatments

Sexual and reproductive history

Cardiopulmonary status

Past or current neurological or neurocognitive disorders or symptoms

Past physical trauma, including head injuries

Past or current endocrinological disease

Past or current infectious disease, including sexually transmitted diseases, HIV, tuberculosis, hepatitis C, and locally endemic infectious diseases such as Lyme disease

Past or current sleep abnormalities, including sleep apnea

Past or current symptoms or conditions associated with significant pain and discomfort

Additional review of systems, as indicated

Family history

Including history of suicidal behaviors or aggressive behaviors in biological relatives

TABLE 2.   Recommended aspects of the initial psychiatric evaluation *(continued)*

Personal and social history

Preferred language and need for an interpreter

Personal/cultural beliefs, sociocultural environment, and cultural explanations of psychiatric illness

Presence of psychosocial stressors (e.g., financial, housing, legal, school/occupational, or interpersonal/relationship problems; lack of social support; painful, disfiguring, or terminal medical illness)

Exposure to physical, sexual, or emotional trauma

Exposure to violence or aggressive behavior, including combat exposure or childhood abuse

Legal or disciplinary consequences of past aggressive behaviors

Examination, including mental status examination

General appearance and nutritional status

Height, weight, and body mass index (BMI)

Vital signs

Skin, including any stigmata of trauma, self-injury, or drug use

Coordination and gait

Involuntary movements or abnormalities of motor tone

Sight and hearing

Speech, including fluency and articulation

Mood, degree of hopelessness, and level of anxiety

Thought content, process, and perceptions, including current hallucinations, delusions, negative symptoms, and insight

Cognition

Current suicidal ideas, suicide plans, and suicide intent, including active or passive thoughts of suicide or death

If current suicidal ideas are present, assess patient's intended course of action if current symptoms worsen; access to suicide methods including firearms; possible motivations for suicide (e.g., attention or reaction from others, revenge, shame, humiliation, delusional guilt, command hallucinations); reasons for living (e.g., sense of responsibility to children or others, religious beliefs); and quality and strength of the therapeutic alliance.

Current aggressive ideas, including thoughts of physical or sexual aggression or homicide

If current aggressive ideas are present, assess specific individuals or groups toward whom patient's homicidal or aggressive ideas or behaviors have been directed in the past or at present; impulsivity, including anger management issues and access to firearms.

Source.   Adapted from American Psychiatric Association 2016a.

et al. 2023; Zimmerman et al. 2022). These biases, stigma, and self-stigma can also influence assessment and diagnosis related to BPD (Klein et al. 2022a; Masland et al. 2023; McKenzie et al. 2022; Stiles et al. 2023). In addition, disparities in assessment and diagnosis based on race or gender identity are common (Denning et al. 2022; Goldhammer et al. 2019; Masland et al. 2023; Olbert et al. 2018; Rodriguez-Seijas et al. 2021; Schwartz and Blankenship 2014; Zimmerman et al. 2022).

Many individuals with BPD will also have had traumatic experiences during their lifetime, such as childhood maltreatment, sexual trauma, or violent victimization (de Aquino Ferreira et al. 2018; Hailes et al. 2019; Porter et al. 2020; Tate et al. 2022). Sensitivity to the impact of these experiences, including use of trauma-informed approaches, can aid in establishing a supportive environment that is conducive to rapport (Burns et al. 2023; Center for Substance Abuse Treatment 2014; Huo et al. 2023; Menschner and Maul 2016; National Council for Mental Wellbeing 2019; Raja et al. 2015;

Rudolph 2021; Saunders et al. 2023; Substance Abuse and Mental Health Services Administration 2014). Depending on the circumstances of the initial evaluation, it may be preferable to defer discussion of prior traumatic experiences until a therapeutic relationship is established or until the setting is more conducive to obtaining detailed information.

Throughout the assessment process, it is important to gain an understanding of the patient's goals, view of the illness, and preferences for treatment. This information will serve as a starting point for person-centered care and shared decision-making with the patient, family, friends, and others involved in the patient's care (Dixon et al. 2016; Hamann and Heres 2019). It will also provide a framework for recovery, which has been defined as "a process of change through which individuals improve their health and wellness, live self-directed lives, and strive to reach their full potential" (Substance Abuse and Mental Health Services Administration 2012, p. 3). Consequently, discussions of goals should be focused beyond symptom relief and may include goals related to schooling, employment, living situation, relationships, leisure activities, and other aspects of functioning and quality of life. Family context and educational factors are particularly crucial to identify when assessing adolescents and emerging adults. Questions about the patient's views may help determine whether the patient is aware of having an illness and assist in understanding the patient's explanations for or experience of their symptoms or distress (Saks 2009). Based on prior treatment experiences, patients may have specific views about such topics as medications, other treatment approaches, mechanical restraints, or involuntary treatment. It is also important to inquire about the patient's strengths and protective factors. For example, they may be able to delineate strategies that have been helpful for them in coping with or managing their symptoms in the past (Cohen et al. 2017). Some patients will have completed a psychiatric advance directive (Murray and Wortzel 2019) and, if so, it will be important to review that with them.

In addition to direct interview, patients may be asked to complete electronic or paper-based forms that ask about psychiatric symptoms or key aspects of the history (American Psychiatric Association 2016a). When available, prior medical records, electronic prescription databases, and input from other treating clinicians can add further details to the history or corroborate information obtained in the interview (American Psychiatric Association 2016a).

People with BPD have heterogeneous relationships with family members, friends, and other individuals. Often, family members, friends, or others in the patient's support network can be an important part of the care team. Such individuals can also serve as valuable sources of collateral information about the reason for evaluation, the patient's past history, and their current symptoms and behavior (American Psychiatric Association 2016a). Input from and engagement of parents, guardians, or other caregivers is particularly important when assessing and treating adolescents and emerging adults.

In other circumstances, a patient may not want a specific family member or other individual to be involved in their care. For example, a patient may wish to avoid burdening a loved one or may have experienced abuse by a particular family member in the past. A patient may also have felt unsupported by family members or others in terms of issues such as their life goals, their gender identity, coping with their BPD symptoms, or other aspects of their lives. For these reasons, the patient's permission is typically obtained before outreach to family, friends, and others in the support network, except in emergent situations to prevent or lessen a serious and imminent threat to the health or safety of the patient or others (American Psychiatric Association 2013b, 2016a; Office for Civil Rights 2017). In addition, under the Health Insurance Portability and Accountability Act of 1996 (HIPAA; Office for Civil Rights 2017), a clinician may listen to information provided by a family member or other involved person, as long as confidential information about the patient is not provided to that individual (American Psychiatric Association 2016a).

The initial evaluation typically begins with the reason the individual is presenting for evaluation. Common concerns in individuals with BPD include anxiety, depression, mood instability, irritability, difficulties with anger, hopelessness, low self-esteem, unstable self-image or sense of self, unstable and intense interpersonal relationships, concerns about real or feared abandonment, suicidal thoughts or attempts, NSSI, other impulsive or self-harming behaviors (e.g., substance use, reckless driving, risky sexual behavior), or harm to others.

As part of the initial evaluation, it is useful to ask about the onset, course, and duration of symptoms. Features common in BPD that can aid in establishing a diagnosis include extreme responses to real or imagined abandonment, sudden shifts in the person's views of others, intense dysphoria, prominent mood reactivity, chronic feelings of emptiness, or intense anger (American Psychiatric Association 2022a). Other illness-driven behaviors, such as self-injurious behavior, may also be present. Specific questions may be needed to identify whether the patient has had transient dissociative experiences, hallucinations, ideas of reference, or persecutory ideas, particularly in periods of stress (American Psychiatric Association 2022a). It is also helpful to determine whether impairments are present in self-functioning (i.e., identity and self-direction) and in interpersonal functioning (i.e., empathy and intimacy) (American Psychiatric Association 2022a).

If the patient has received treatment previously, it is important to ask about a broad range of treatments and other approaches used to address the patient's symptoms and functioning and to specifically ask about the full range of treatment settings (e.g., outpatient, partial hospitalization, inpatient) and approaches or aspects of the therapeutic relationships that the patient has found helpful or problematic (American Psychiatric Association 2016a; Bachelor 2013; Barnicot et al. 2022; de Freixo Ferreira et al. 2023; Woodbridge et al. 2023). For example, prompting may be needed to learn information about the patient's experiences with psychotherapies (e.g., dialectical behavior therapy [DBT], cognitive-behavioral therapy [CBT], mentalization-based treatment [MBT], transference-focused psychotherapy [TFP], schema-focused therapy [SFT], dynamic deconstructive psychotherapy [DDP], other psychodynamic therapies, couples or family therapy, supportive therapy) as well as their formats, frequencies, and durations. A patient may believe that they have not responded to a specific type of psychotherapy, but the fidelity to key treatment principles (as described in the "Implementation" section of Statement 5) may have been limited or the treatment intensity or duration may have been insufficient. The formats and focus of the different psychotherapies may be a good fit for some individuals but not for others; for example, some but not all patients do well with the structure of homework assignments, some prefer individual treatment to groups, and some prefer insight-oriented approaches to skills-based approaches (Woodbridge et al. 2023). With medications, information about the specific medication, duration of treatment, formulation, route, and dosage are important to obtain. Specific questions may be needed on long-acting injectable (LAI) medications (e.g., antipsychotics, naltrexone, buprenorphine) or implants (e.g., buprenorphine, contraceptive agents), over-the-counter medications, herbal products, or nutritional supplements because these medications may be overlooked by patients and are less likely to be included in pharmacy databases and patients' lists of active medications. Experimental treatments such as psilocybin and ketamine are increasingly available. Other interventions can include substance use treatments, neuromodulatory therapies (e.g., electroconvulsive therapy [ECT], transcranial magnetic stimulation [TMS]), court-ordered treatment, treatment while incarcerated, 12-step programs, self-help groups, culture-based approaches, spiritual healers, and complementary or alternative treatment approaches. For each specific type of intervention that the patient has received, it is important to learn more about their response (including tolerability, changes in quality of life, level of functioning, symptom response/remission, and persistence of improvement) as well as their engagement in therapy and degree of adherence.

A thorough history is also important for identifying the presence of co-occurring psychiatric conditions or physical disorders that need to be addressed in treatment planning (American Psychiatric Association 2016a; Firth et al. 2019). Substance use and SUDs are common in individuals with BPD (Grant et al. 2008; Trull et al. 2018), and some individuals with BPD may use substances to cope with their emotional distress or help regulate their emotions. Therefore, a substance use history will be valuable in determining whether the individual uses tobacco, marijuana, or other substances such as alcohol, caffeine, nicotine, cocaine, opioids, sedative-hypnotic agents, stimulants, 3,4-methylenedioxymethamphetamine (MDMA), solvents, androgenic steroids, hallucinogens, ketamine, or synthetic substances (e.g., "bath salts," K2, Spice). The route by which substances are used (e.g., ingestion, smoking, vaping, intranasal, intravenous) and the frequency and circumstances of use are also important to document.

In addition to SUDs, other common co-occurring psychiatric conditions in individuals with BPD include MDD, bipolar disorder, PTSD, anxiety disorders, eating disorders, ADHD, and other personality disorders (Choi-Kain et al. 2022; Friborg et al. 2014; Geluk Rouwhorst et al. 2023; Grant et al. 2016; Gunderson et al. 2014; Keuroghlian et al. 2015; Leichsenring et al. 2011; Lenzenweger et al. 2007; McDermid et al. 2015; McGlashan et al. 2000; Miller et al. 2022; Momen et al. 2022; Philipsen et al. 2008; Santo et al. 2022; Tate et al. 2022; Trull et al. 2018; Zanarini et al. 2004a, 2010, 2019; Zimmerman et al. 2017). Individuals with BPD may also have physical health conditions, sleep disturbances, or chronic pain that need to be considered in assessing functioning and developing a plan of treatment (Doering 2019; El-Gabalawy et al. 2010; Heath et al. 2018b; Kalira et al. 2013; Sansone and Sansone 2012; Vanek et al. 2021; Winsper et al. 2017). Prior head trauma or other brain abnormalities (e.g., due to anoxic injury) can contribute to impulsivity or emotional dysregulation (McHugo et al. 2017).

The psychosocial history reviews the stages of the patient's life and may include attention to perinatal events, delays in developmental milestones, disruptive behavioral disorders in childhood, childhood maltreatment (including neglect or emotional, physical, or sexual abuse), academic history and performance (including a history of being bullied, learning difficulties, special education interventions, or disciplinary actions), occupational history (including military history), legal history, and identification of major life events (e.g., adoption or foster care, family separation, parental loss, divorce, migration history, sexual trauma, other traumatic experiences) and psychosocial stressors (e.g., financial, housing, legal, school/occupational, or interpersonal/relationship problems; childcare or other caregiving responsibilities; lack of social support; trauma related to racial/ethnic discrimination; discrimination or trauma related to LGBTQ+ identity; painful, disfiguring, or terminal medical illness; other social determinants of health) (American Psychiatric Association 2016a; Barnhill 2014; MacKinnon et al. 2016; Smith et al. 2019). Information on the patient's gender identity and pronouns are also important to elicit.

Individuals may have received disability-related income support, supported employment, or accommodations related to disability in academic, workplace, or other settings. Such accommodations are important to be aware of because they can help promote functioning and enhance integration into the community. If patients are eligible for disability-related income support, supported employment, or disability-related accommodations but have not received them, this will also be relevant to treatment planning. Furthermore, inquiring into an individual's accommodation history can serve as a starting point for discussion around accessibility needs during treatment and ensuring that these are met.

The patient's history of interpersonal relationships, including family and intimate relationships, is particularly essential to obtain. Such relationships can be supportive and helpful, or they can be unstable or intense in individuals with BPD. The patient's current and prior degree of interpersonal functioning (including in academic, occupational, social, and family roles, such as parenting) is similarly vital to the history and subsequent treatment planning. Assessment of interpersonal functioning should take developmental considerations into account, particularly in adolescents and emerging adults. Information about the patient's family constellation and other persons who provide support serves as a foundation for working collaboratively with the patient and their support network. A family health history is also important in identifying family members who have a history of personality disorder, particularly BPD or BPD traits, as well as the presence of SUDs, other psychiatric disorders, or suicidal behaviors in the family.

The patient's cultural history is similarly integral to understanding them and developing an effective plan of treatment. In addition to emphasizing relationships, both familial and nonfamilial, it also delineates the role of important cultural, spiritual, and religious beliefs and practices in the patient's life (Aggarwal and Lewis-Fernández 2015; American Psychiatric Association 2022b;

Lewis-Fernández et al. 2016). The Cultural Formulation Interview (American Psychiatric Association 2022b) provides a framework for obtaining this information as part of the evaluation. Clinicians should be especially careful to avoid cultural bias when applying the diagnostic criteria and evaluating sexual behavior, expressions of emotion, suspiciousness, or impulsiveness, which may have different norms in different cultures or subcultures. Individuals from different cultures or with different spiritual or religious beliefs may also have different views of roles among family members and intimate partners as well as different views of and knowledge about health and mental health, including diagnoses, treatments, attitudes, and beliefs toward the patient's health and mental health issues.

The mental status examination is an essential part of the initial assessment. A full delineation of the mental status examination is beyond the scope of this document, and detailed information on conducting the examination is available elsewhere (American Psychiatric Association 2016a; Barnhill 2014; MacKinnon et al. 2016; Smith et al. 2019; Strub and Black 2000). In addition, for individuals with possible BPD, risk assessment is particularly important. It is crucial to identify past and current risks to self (e.g., suicidal ideas, methods, plans, and intent; NSSI; suicide attempts, including interrupted and aborted suicide attempts) and risks to others (e.g., aggressive or homicidal thoughts, statements, or behaviors). Information gathered and synthesized as part of the history and mental status examination will help identify modifiable risk factors for suicidal or aggressive behaviors that can serve as targets of intervention when constructing a plan of treatment. Inquiring about the patient's degree of insight and judgment, as discussed earlier, also provides information relevant to risk assessment, treatment outcomes, and adherence (Mintz et al. 2003; Mohamed et al. 2009).

Statement 2 – Quantitative Measures

APA *suggests* **(2C)** that the initial psychiatric evaluation of a patient with possible borderline personality disorder include a quantitative measure to identify and determine the severity of symptoms and impairments of functioning that may be a focus of treatment.

Implementation

Several rating scales are available that have been used to identify and determine the severity of symptoms of BPD. Although rating scales have primarily been used in research contexts, they can also be used clinically to complement other aspects of the screening and assessment process (American Psychiatric Association 2016a).

Use of rating scales can aid treatment planning in several ways. Such measures provide a structured, replicable way to document the patient's baseline symptoms. They also can help to determine which symptoms should be the target of intervention on the basis of factors such as frequency of occurrence, magnitude, or impact on the patient's functioning, well-being, and quality of life. As treatment proceeds, use of quantitative measures allows more precise tracking of whether psychotherapies or other treatments are having their intended effect or whether a shift in the treatment plan is needed (Lewis et al. 2019). The exact frequency of measures depends on clinical circumstances. Nevertheless, it is preferable to use a consistent approach to quantitative measurement for a given patient because each rating scale defines and measures symptoms differently. In addition, patients' ratings can be compared with family members' impressions of treatment effects to clarify the longitudinal course of the patient's illness.

When rating scales are used, they should always be implemented in a way that supports developing and maintaining the therapeutic relationship with the patient. Often, patient-rated scales are less time-consuming to administer than clinician-rated scales or structured or semistructured interviews. The use of anchored, self-rated scales with criteria to assess the severity and frequency of symptoms can also help patients become more informed self-observers. In addition, they provide important insights into the patient's experience that support person-centered care. Reviewing scale results with the patient can help foster a collaborative dialogue about progress toward symptom improvement, functioning gains, and recovery goals. Such a review may help clinicians, patients, families, and other support persons recognize that improvement is occurring or, conversely, identify issues that need further attention.

If more than one quantitative measure is being used, it is important to minimize duplication of questions and avoid overwhelming the patient with an excessive number of scales to complete. Optimal scale properties (e.g., sensitivity, specificity) differ depending on the desired purpose(s) for using the scale in a given patient. In addition, when choosing among available quantitative measures, the psychometric properties (e.g., scale validity, reliability)[1] and the objectives for using the scale (e.g., screening, documenting baseline symptoms, ongoing monitoring) should be considered. Assessments of scale properties are typically conducted cross-sectionally, however; therefore, less information may be available about longitudinal use.

A number of factors can affect the interpretation of quantitative measures. For example, some scales ask the patient to rate symptoms over several weeks, which can reduce their ability to detect changes in symptoms. This can be particularly problematic in acute care settings, where treatment adjustments and symptom improvement can occur quickly. Other symptom-based quantitative measures focus either on symptom frequency over the observation period or on symptom severity. Although these features often increase or decrease in parallel, that is not invariably the case. Quantitative measures that ask the patient to consider both symptom frequency and severity can also make the findings difficult to interpret.

It is also possible for rating scales to introduce biases into the assessment process. Factors such as comorbid illnesses, age, language, race, ethnicity, sex/gender, cultural background, literacy, and health literacy are often inadequately addressed during rating scale development. These factors and others can affect patients' interpretation of questions. Thus, the answers to questions and the summative scores on quantitative measures need to be interpreted in the context of the rating scale's properties and the patient's clinical presentation.

The type and extent of quantitative measures used will also be determined by the clinical setting, the time available for evaluation, the urgency of the situation, the availability of validated rating scales in the patient's primary language, and the patient's age. In adolescents, for example, self-report scales and ratings from parents/guardians and teachers can provide helpful information (De Los Reyes et al. 2015). In some clinical contexts, such as a planned outpatient assessment, patients may be asked to complete electronic- or paper-based quantitative measures, either prior to the visit or on arrival at the office (Allen et al. 2009; Harding et al. 2011). Between or prior to visits, electronic approaches (e.g., mobile phone applications, clinical registries, patient portal sites in electronic health records) may also facilitate obtaining quantitative measurements (Lewis et al. 2019; Palmier-Claus et al. 2012; Wang et al. 2018). In other clinical contexts, such as acute inpatient settings, electronic modes of data capture may be more challenging. As an alternative, printed versions of scales may be completed by the patient (or a proxy) or administered by the clinician. In emergency settings, use of a quantitative rating scale may need to be postponed until the acute crisis has subsided or until the patient's clinical status permits a detailed examination. Furthermore, some patients may have difficulty completing self-report instruments due to severe symptoms, co-occurring psychiatric conditions, low health literacy, reading difficulties, or cognitive impairment (Harding et al. 2011; Narrow et al. 2013; Valenstein et al. 2009; Zimmerman et al. 2011).

Although recommending a particular measure is outside the scope of this practice guideline, a number of objective, quantitative rating scales are available for monitoring the symptoms and fea-

---

[1]Although this discussion of rating scales uses the words "reliability" and "validity" as applying to a scale, as is common in the literature, it should be noted that it is only possible to assess the reliability of test scores (not the test itself) and to assess the validity of interpretations that are made from scale scores (American Educational Research Association, American Psychological Association, and National Council for Measurement in Education 2014).

tures of BPD. The 23-item version of the Borderline Symptom List (BSL-23), which is condensed from the 93-item version (Bohus et al. 2007; Central Institute of Mental Health 2020), is a freely available self-report scale that assesses 23 feelings and experiences typically reported by BPD patients (Kleindienst et al. 2020). Individuals are asked to describe the extent to which they experienced a particular item in the past week based on a scale from 0 (not at all) to 4 (very strong) (Kleindienst et al. 2020). The BSL-23, similar to the BSL-93, was found to have high internal consistency, good sensitivity to the effects of treatment, and an ability to discriminate BPD from other psychiatric diagnoses (Bohus et al. 2009). In addition, symptom severity as measured by the BSL-23 appears to correlate with treatment seeking, as well as with the presence of a BPD diagnosis (Kleindienst et al. 2020).

The Borderline Evaluation of Severity Over Time (BEST) is another freely available self-report scale that focuses on the degree to which a symptom interfered with life in the past week and on idealization/devaluation shifts in relationships (Pfohl et al. 2009). In addition, the BEST includes two anger-related items, two abandonment-related items, one item for other BPD criteria, and an item for suicidal ideation (Pfohl et al. 2009). It is reported to have high internal consistency and moderate test-retest reliability (Pfohl et al. 2009).

For adolescents, the 11-item Borderline Personality Features Scale for Children includes self-report and parent-report versions (Sharp et al. 2011, 2014; Vanwoerden et al. 2019; Wall et al. 2019).

The self-report version of the Zanarini Rating Scale for Borderline Personality Disorder (ZAN-BPD; Zanarini et al. 2015) is developed from and organized and scored similarly to the interview-based version of the ZAN-BPD (Zanarini et al. 2003). Both versions of the scale require the author's permission for use, are based on the nine items in the DSM-IV criteria for BPD, and include anchored ratings on a five-point scale from 0 (no symptoms) to 4 (severe symptoms). The scores for each item can be summed to yield a total score, or scores can be calculated for four symptom domains: affective, cognitive, impulsive, and interpersonal (Zanarini et al. 1990). Alternatively, the self-report version of the rating scale can be formatted with Yes/No answers to questions for use as a screening measure. Both versions of the ZAN-BPD showed adequate sensitivity to change at 7–10 days (Zanarini et al. 2015). In addition, scores of the self-report version of the ZAN-BPD showed high convergent validity with scores based on the interview version of the scale as well as good internal consistency and excellent same day test-retest reliability (Zanarini et al. 2015).

The Difficulty in Emotional Regulation Scale (DERS; Gratz and Roemer 2004) is another self-report scale that has been used clinically and in research studies of individuals with BPD. It is freely available and consists of 36 items rated from 1 (almost never) to 5 (almost always) that address six domains: nonacceptance of negative emotions, inability to engage in goal-directed behaviors when distressed, difficulties controlling impulsive behaviors when distressed, limited access to emotion regulation strategies perceived as effective, lack of emotional awareness, and lack of emotional clarity. The psychometric properties of the DERS have been noted to be improved by removing the scale items related to awareness (Hallion et al. 2018; Lee et al. 2016). However, in other respects, the DERS scores generally have good internal consistency and construct validity in adolescents as well as adults (Fowler et al. 2014; Gratz and Roemer 2004; Neumann et al. 2010; Ritschel et al. 2015). In addition, it shows changes with treatment (Gratz et al. 2014; McCauley et al. 2018). Several shortened versions of the DERS are available: the DERS-18 (Victor and Klonsky 2016), the DERS-16 (Bjureberg et al. 2016), the DERS-8 (Penner et al. 2022), and the DERS-SF (Kaufman et al. 2016). Results of the shortened versions correlated with findings on the full 36-item scale. Two studies that compared the original 36-item DERS with the DERS-18, DERS-16, and DERS-SF did not find any of these shortened versions to be superior to the others (Hallion et al. 2018; Skutch et al. 2019).

Self-harm, including suicide attempts and NSSI, is common among individuals with BPD (Grilo and Udo 2021; Yen et al. 2021; Zanarini et al. 2008). Although many of the rating scales for BPD symptoms include items related to self-harm, multiple scales exist that provide more detailed information about self-harming behaviors (Latimer et al. 2012; Sansone and Sansone 2010). One example of such a scale is the Deliberate Self-Harm Inventory (DSHI; Gratz 2001), which is a freely available 17-item self-report tool with good test-retest reliability and construct validity (Fliege et al. 2006; Gratz 2001). In addition to noting which self-harming behaviors are present and their frequency, information from the scale can be transformed into a continuous variable by summing the frequency scores for each item (Gratz and Gunderson 2006). Another scale, the Inventory of Statements About Self-injury, is aimed at assessing the patient's perspective on interpersonal and intrapersonal functions of non-suicidal self-injurious behaviors (Klonsky and Glenn 2009).

The Level of Personality Functioning Scale-Brief Form 2.0 (LPFS-BF) is aimed at assessing personality function more broadly, consistent with the AMPD (Hutsebaut et al. 2016; Weekers et al. 2019). It is freely available and consists of 12 statements rated as "very false or often false," "sometimes or somewhat false," "sometimes or somewhat true," or "very true or often true." Factor analysis suggested that the LPFS-BF evaluates two domains: self-functioning and interpersonal functioning (Weekers et al. 2019). In addition, there was high sensitivity to change at 3 months of treatment, adding to the evidence that LPFS-BF scores are indicative of personality functioning (Le Corff et al. 2022; Weekers et al. 2019).

Other self-report rating scales of relevance to individuals with a personality disorder have been reviewed in detail by the International Consortium for Health Outcomes Measurement (ICHOM), a multidisciplinary international working group that conducted a systematic review and subsequent Delphi process to develop a standard set of outcome measures for individuals with personality disorders (Prevolnik Rupel et al. 2021).

Because reductions in symptoms can occur despite significant impairments in quality of life or functioning (Gunderson et al. 2011; Niesten et al. 2016), rating scales that assess these latter domains can also provide helpful information. One example of a scale that can be utilized to assess quality of life is the WHOQOL-BREF scale (Skevington et al. 2004; WHOQOL Group 1998; http://depts.washington.edu/seaqol/WHOQOL-BREF), developed by the World Health Organization. For assessing functioning difficulties due to health and mental health conditions, DSM-5 (American Psychiatric Association 2013a) includes the 36-item self- and proxy-administered versions of the World Health Organization Disability Schedule 2.0 (WHODAS 2.0; American Psychiatric Association 2013c; Üstün et al. 2010). Other options for assessing functioning include the Social and Occupational Functioning Assessment Scale (SOFAS; American Psychiatric Association 2000) and the Personal and Social Performance scale (Morosini et al. 2000). Several versions of Patient-Reported Outcomes Measurement Information System (PROMIS) scales, which address social roles and functioning, are also available (www.healthmeasures.net/explore-measurement-systems/promis).

Statement 3 – Treatment Planning

APA *recommends* (**1C**) that a patient with borderline personality disorder have a documented, comprehensive, and person-centered treatment plan.

Implementation

Overview of Treatment Planning

When treating individuals with BPD, a person-centered treatment plan should be developed, documented in the medical record, and updated at appropriate intervals. Whenever possible, development and updating of the treatment plan should be done in a collaborative fashion with the patient. When treating an adolescent, parents or other involved caregivers will be crucial to engage when creating a treatment plan. Although patients' relationships with family members can be heterogeneous, many adults will welcome involvement of family members and others (Cohen et al. 2013; Lamont and Dickens 2021). Input from these individuals can be vital in developing a full picture of the patient (as discussed in Statement 1) as well as in formulating and implementing a person-centered treatment plan. If the patient is also receiving care from another health professional, for BPD or for other conditions, communication with those individuals is essential.

A person-centered treatment plan can be recorded as part of an evaluation note or progress note and does not need to adhere to a defined development process (e.g., face-to-face multidisciplinary team meeting) or format (e.g., time-specified goals and objectives). Depending on the urgency of the initial clinical presentation and the availability of other sources of information, the initial treatment plan may need to be augmented over several visits as more details of history and treatment response are obtained. When adapting treatment to the needs of the individual patient, the treatment plan may also need to be tailored on the basis of developmental, sociocultural, or dimensional aspects of personality pathology, with an aim of enhancing quality of life or aspects of functioning (e.g., social, academic, occupational). Adjustments to the treatment plan will occur throughout the course of treatment as symptoms or presenting concerns change and as the clinical formulation evolves.

The overarching aims of treatment are 1) to promote and maintain recovery, 2) to maximize quality of life and adaptive functioning, 3) to reduce or eliminate symptoms, including self-injurious and suicidal behaviors, and 4) to address developmental considerations and co-occurring disorders in the context of BPD treatment. To achieve these aims and inform treatment planning, it is crucial to identify the patient's aspirations, goals for treatment, and treatment-related preferences. For patients who have completed a psychiatric advance directive (Kemp et al. 2015; Shields et al. 2014; Wilder et al. 2010), wellness recovery action plan (Copeland 2000), or individualized crisis prevention or safety plan (Stanley and Brown 2012; Stanley et al. 2018), these documents will be important to review with the patient when crafting a person-centered approach to care. When developing an individual treatment plan, the clinician should explain and discuss the range of treatments available for the patient's condition, the modalities being recommended, and the associated rationale for having selected them. As part of the discussion, the patient's views of the proposed treatment will be elicited and the plan can be modified, to the extent feasible, to incorporate their views and preferences.

Elements of the Treatment Plan

Depending on the clinical circumstances and input from the patient and others, a comprehensive and person-centered treatment plan will typically delineate treatments aimed at improving functioning, reducing symptoms, and addressing the core personality features of BPD. If co-occurring psychiatric symptoms or disorders are present, it is important to identify them and to incorporate appropriate interventions into the treatment plan. Psychotherapeutic approaches will be at the core of the treatment plan for BPD (see Guideline Statement 5), but medications may also be appropriate to use, typically on a limited basis (see Guideline Statements 6 through 8).

Other elements of the treatment plan often include the following:

- Identifying needs for additional evaluation
  - History or mental status examination
  - Physical examination (either by the evaluating clinician or by another health professional)
  - Laboratory testing, imaging, electrocardiography (ECG), or other clinical studies (if indicated on the basis of the history, examination, and planned treatments)
- Determining the most appropriate treatment setting
- Providing psychoeducation about BPD and approaches to treatment
- Addressing barriers to adherence
- Collaborating with other treating clinicians
- Involving family members, other caregivers, and other individuals in the patient's support network
- Delineating plans for addressing risks of harm to self or others, if present
- Addressing co-occurring disorders, if present
- Incorporating goals of treatment related to culturally sensitive care, as well as psychosocial con-

siderations such as school or employment, past or current adversity, or interpersonal, family, or intimate relationships

Determining a Treatment Setting

When determining a treatment setting, considerations for individuals with BPD are similar to those for individuals with other diagnoses. Thus, in general, patients should be cared for in the least restrictive setting that is likely to be safe and to allow for effective treatment of BPD and co-occurring conditions. Often, outpatient treatment will be the appropriate setting of care. When a patient requires more monitoring or assistance than is available in routine outpatient care, programs that provide an intermediate level of care (e.g., intensive outpatient programs, partial hospital programs, residential treatment programs) may be indicated. Although evidence is limited, assertive community treatment has occasionally been used for individuals with BPD who have complex health and social service needs, particularly when treatment adherence has been challenging (Grambal et al. 2017; Horvitz-Lennon et al. 2009b).

Indications for hospitalization usually include the patient posing a serious threat of harm to self or others or being unable to care for themselves and needing constant supervision or support as a result. Other possible indications for hospitalization include psychiatric or other medical problems that make outpatient treatment unsafe or ineffective and that warrant initial inpatient stabilization to promote reduction of acute symptoms and permit engagement in treatment. If inpatient care is deemed essential, efforts should be made to hospitalize patients voluntarily. If hospitalization is deemed essential but is not accepted voluntarily by the patient, state or jurisdictional requirements for involuntary hospitalization should be followed.

Determination of treatment setting will also require weighing the pluses and minuses of possible settings to identify the optimal location for care. For example, hospitalization can have benefits in terms of safety but add to financial burdens; disrupt school, work, or caregiving responsibilities; or be upsetting for patients due to repeated hospitalizations (Comtois and Carmel 2016) or to negative experiences with inpatient care (Stapleton and Wright 2019). In most circumstances, management of the patient on an inpatient psychiatric service in collaboration with consultants of other medical specialties will be optimal. However, individuals with BPD who have other significant health issues may need significant medical or surgical interventions or monitoring that are not typically available on a psychiatric inpatient service. Under such circumstances, the patient will likely be better served on a general hospital unit or in an intensive care setting with input from consultation-liaison psychiatrists and education and supervision of staff to help them engage with the patient in a therapeutic and non-judgmental fashion.

Establishing and Maintaining a Therapeutic Framework and Alliance

The therapeutic relationship is an essential ingredient in the treatment of patients with BPD (Bender 2005; Rudge et al. 2020) and for mental health treatment in general (Baier et al. 2020; Frank and Frank 1993; Oldham 2022b; Stubbe 2018). Because patients with BPD may have difficulty developing and sustaining trusting relationships, establishing and strengthening the therapeutic alliance will generally be a focus of treatment from the initial session (Culina et al. 2023). Although the underpinnings of the therapeutic alliance vary, clinicians are expected to offer understanding, responsiveness, explanations for treatment interventions, undistracted attention, and respectful, validating, and compassionate attitudes, with judicious feedback to patients that can help the patients develop self-efficacy and attain their goals. In addition to interactions with the treating clinician or treatment team, the therapeutic alliance can also be affected by the patient's prior experiences, including those related to biases and health disparities (e.g., related to race, ethnicity, sexual orientation, or sex/gender) (Maharaj et al. 2021; Spengler et al. 2016; Sue et al. 2007).

At the outset of treatment, it is important to establish a clear and explicit treatment framework with which the patient agrees (Sledge et al. 2014). Although this process is generally applicable to the treatment of all patients, regardless of diagnosis, such an agreement is particularly important for patients with BPD and can serve as a model for healthy boundaries in other aspects of the patient's life. As part of this treatment framework, patients and clinicians should establish agreements about the goals of treatment sessions (e.g., symptom reduction, personal growth, improvement in functioning), ways to facilitate these goals (e.g., reporting on such issues as conflicts, dysfunction, and impending life changes; completing homework between sessions; developing an individualized safety plan), and what role each is expected to perform to achieve these goals. Although some therapeutic approaches incorporate specific criteria that would lead treatment to be discontinued, it is always important to emphasize these aspects of the treatment framework that will help contribute to treatment success. In addition, it is essential for patients and clinicians to work toward establishing agreements about 1) when, where, and with what frequency sessions will be held; 2) notification of planned or urgent session cancellations or delays in keeping appointments; 3) the fee, billing, and payment schedule; 4) clarification of the clinician's after-hours availability; and 5) a plan for crisis management, which may include a coordinated plan for patients to have intersession access to the treatment team. Furthermore, it is important to review expectations if emergency care is needed. Mechanisms for emergency department staff to reach and communicate with the treatment team are equally important when a patient is in crisis.

To adhere to a framework for successful treatment, clinicians often need to communicate with patients about realistic limits while simultaneously addressing patient concerns. In communicating limits, the clinician should recognize that an excessive focus on limits may overshadow treatment goals and compromise the therapeutic alliance. Rather, the focus should be on preventing harm to the patient, maintaining appropriate boundaries to facilitate treatment, and fostering open communication about the patient's experience in treatment. For example, clinicians may need to reiterate aspects related to payment, times when they can be available to the patient, clinical coverage during vacations, or plans for dealing with phone calls or crises (Epstein 1994; Gabbard and Wilkinson 2000; Skodol and Oldham 2021). Clinicians may also need to address specific patient behaviors that would be disruptive to the therapeutic relationship or that would suggest a need for treatment plan revisions. For example, patients may be reluctant to disclose self-harming behaviors, yet recognizing that these behaviors are occurring could lead the clinician to a greater understanding of the patient's internal experiences. In addition, patients, family members, or others involved in the patient's care may need to raise concerns about factors that could rupture the therapeutic relationship (e.g., sudden changes in the clinician's schedule; perceived biases in the clinician's attitude or interactions; negative experiences with the clinician, other treatment team members, administrative staff members, or other group therapy participants). In discussing such concerns, the clinician should remain nonjudgmental while gaining an understanding of the patient's experience.

The intensity of the patient's emotional experience and the behaviors that are part of BPD can also evoke various emotional reactions (i.e., countertransference) in clinicians ranging from warmth and empathy to desires to "rescue" the patient to negative feelings (e.g., frustration, anger) (Bhola and Mehrotra 2021). If not recognized by the clinician, such emotional reactions can impact clinical decision-making in ways that are not in the patient's best interest. Team consultation and supervision are important avenues for understanding these emotional responses and the perspectives of different clinicians so that treatment is not adversely affected. If treatment is discontinued, whether by the patient or the clinician, attention should be given to its timing and to transfer of care (American Medical Association Code of Medical Ethics 2023a). If the treatment termination process is unusually difficult or complex, a consultation with another clinician should be considered.

Even when the treatment framework has been developed and agreed to at the start of treatment, situations can arise in which the boundaries of the framework become blurred or are crossed (Bender 2005; Gutheil 2005). Certain situations (e.g., practicing in a small community, rural area, or military setting) may complicate the task of maintaining treatment boundaries (Sederer et al. 1998). The advent of the internet and social media has introduced additional challenges (Gabbard et al. 2011). Nevertheless, it is always the clinician's responsibility to monitor and sustain the treatment framework. Furthermore, clinicians should be proactive in exploring the meaning of any boundary crossing—whether originating from their own behavior or that of the patient—and restate their expectations about the treatment boundaries and their rationale (Bender 2005; Gutheil 2005). Clinicians should also be alert to their own feelings toward the patient and any deviations from their usual way of practicing that may signal a risk of boundary violations (e.g., appointments at unusual hours, longer-than-usual appointments, doing special favors for the patient, developing a personal friendship outside of the professional situation) (Gutheil 2005). In such circumstances, consultation, personal psychotherapy, or both may be warranted. Sexual interactions between a clinician and a patient are always unethical and, in most jurisdictions, a reportable event that can affect continued licensure (Gutheil 2005; MacIntyre and Appel 2020). If this type of boundary violation occurs, the clinician should immediately refer the patient to another clinician.

Strategies to Promote Adherence

Adherence with treatment is a crucial aspect of achieving therapeutic benefit, yet clinical studies of BPD typically have significant dropout rates (Barnicot et al. 2011; Iliakis et al. 2021). Thus, strategies to promote adherence are always important to consider when developing a patient-centered treatment plan. Adherence will generally be aided by obtaining patient input, engaging in shared decision-making as part of treatment planning, and developing a collaborative therapeutic alliance (Barnicot et al. 2022; de Freixo Ferreira et al. 2023). In youth, one study suggests that youth-oriented case management and psychiatric care focused on BPD is associated with better adherence and treatment retention than general youth-oriented care models (Chanen et al. 2022). Some potential factors that can influence adherence may become evident during the initial evaluation or early sessions. These include difficulties in prior therapeutic relationships, ineffectiveness of prior treatment, viewing treatment as unnecessary, perceptions of stigma about needing treatment (including self-stigma), prior difficulties with adherence, cultural or family beliefs about illness or treatment, lack of support from significant others for treatment, or the presence of co-occurring conditions (e.g., depression; alcohol, cannabis, other SUDs). Other common issues with adherence to treatment include financial barriers (e.g., cost, lack of insurance or underinsurance), difficulties scheduling visits around work or school schedules, limited geographical availability or accessibility of services, or issues with transportation or with childcare. When medications are part of the treatment plan, many of the same elements apply (e.g., cost, lack of perceived need for treatment, concerns about prior treatment experiences or stigma). In addition, patients may have concerns about side effects (e.g., weight gain, sexual dysfunction) or difficulty with managing complex regimens (e.g., due to frequency of doses, number of medications) (Anderson et al. 2020; Kardas et al. 2013; Nieuwlaat et al. 2014; Peh et al. 2021). These potential contributors to nonadherence can be explored proactively or be reassessed if adherence difficulties develop. Addressing these barriers as part of the treatment plan requires active collaboration and problem-solving between the clinician and the patient, often with input from the patient's family and others involved in the patient's life. With adolescents, involvement of parents, family members, and other caregivers is critical.

Using Peer-Support Programs to Enhance Care

Peer-support programs have been used in SUD treatment programs (Substance Abuse and Mental Health Services Administration 2022), as well as in mental health treatment programs (Høgh Egmose et al. 2023; Mirbahaeddin and Chreim 2022) more broadly. Although research on peer support programs has been limited, available evidence suggests that they may have small positive effects on anxiety and personal recovery (Høgh Egmose et al. 2023). Peer support can also be used to complement, but not replace, other treatment approaches in various settings and formats (e.g., individual, group, in-person, online) (Emotions Matter 2023b; Høgh Egmose et al. 2023; Mirbahaeddin and Chreim 2022; Substance Abuse and Mental Health Services Administration 2022). In patients with BPD, peer support may help individuals feel less isolated, more understood, and hopeful and may assist them in developing coping skills with input from the perspective of someone with lived experience (Barr et al. 2020, 2022). When peer support is used as part of the treatment plan, it is important to have a specific framework or structure in place (e.g., as with the peer support groups provided by Emotions Matter 2023b). If peer support services are integrated into hospital-based or outpatient-based treatment programs, other implementation issues should be considered to optimize benefits and to avoid potential harms for the patient and the peer support worker (e.g., role definitions and boundaries, supervision, privacy of patient health records, relationships with team members; Mirbahaeddin and Chreim 2022).

Coordinating the Treatment Effort

Treatment of BPD can be provided by a single clinician performing multiple tasks or by multiple clinicians performing separate treatment tasks. Treatment by multiple clinicians has potential advantages but can contribute to fragmentation of care. Consequently, when a team-based approach to treatment is used, ongoing coordination of the overall treatment plan needs to be ensured through clear role definitions, plans for management of crises, and regular communication among the clinicians and the patient. Often, family members and other caregivers will also be involved in care coordination, and this is particularly crucial in the treatment of adolescents. Communication and coordination of care may also be needed with primary care or specialty care clinicians who are addressing the patient's physical health needs.

When treatment is provided by multiple clinicians, divisiveness or polarization among treatment team members can be associated with the tendency for idealization and devaluation of others (i.e., "splitting") that occurs as a part of BPD. It is the responsibility of the treatment team to manage such issues if they occur, recognize the heightened need for intentional communication, and enhance coordination among involved clinicians to ensure that therapeutic decision-making is not compromised. For this reason, many treatments for BPD are explicit in defining roles and relationships among treatment team members.

Addressing Risks for Suicidal and Aggressive Behavior

General Aspects of Risk Assessment

Identifying risk factors and estimating risks for suicidal and aggressive behaviors are essential parts of psychiatric evaluation (American Psychiatric Association 2016a; described in detail in the "Implementation" section of Statement 1). Despite identification of these risk factors, it is not possible to predict whether a patient will engage in aggressive behaviors or attempt or die by suicide. However, when an increased risk for such behaviors is present, it is important that the treatment plan identifies the optimal setting of care and implements approaches to target and reduce modifiable risk factors. Although demographic and historical risk factors are static, potentially modifiable risk factors may include poor adherence, co-occurring symptoms (e.g., depression, hopelessness, hostility, impulsivity, sleep disturbance), or co-occurring diagnoses (e.g., depression, alcohol use disorder [AUD], other SUDs, physical health conditions). Life events that may increase risk in a patient include traumatic experiences, disrupted relationships, perceived failures at school or work, or discrimination experienced in relation to race, ethnicity, or sex/gender. Risk may be reduced by increased monitoring or more intensive services during periods of increased risk (e.g., with significant psychosocial crises, during incarceration, subsequent to hospital discharge). With adolescents, and often with patients of other ages, involvement of family members or other caregivers can be helpful in strengthening social support networks and providing collateral information that is relevant to risk assessment (Mammen et al. 2020).

Risk for Suicide and Suicidal Behaviors

Although suicidal ideation does not occur in all patients with BPD (Zimmerman and Becker 2023), many individuals with BPD will experience suicidal ideation at some point in their lifetime. It is estimated that self-injurious behavior occurs in more than 90% of individuals with BPD, with suicide attempts in approximately 75% and suicide death in 3%–10% (Black et al. 2004; Cipriano et al.

2017; Goodman et al. 2017; Grilo and Udo 2021; Kjær et al. 2020; Leichsenring et al. 2011; Links et al. 2013; Machado et al. 2022; Paris 2019; Temes et al. 2019; Yen et al. 2021; Zanarini et al. 2008). Managing suicide risk in individuals with BPD can be challenging for several reasons. For the patient, suicidal thoughts are associated with distressing internal experiences that may include feelings of hopelessness, failure, loss of control, or harsh self-criticism (Berg et al. 2017, 2020; Gaily-Luoma et al. 2022; Schechter et al. 2019). In addition, because patients with BPD may have difficulty forming stable interpersonal relationships, it can be difficult for them to work collaboratively in treatment to reduce their risk of serious self-harm or suicide. Furthermore, many patients with BPD have ongoing risk factors for suicide (e.g., prior suicide attempts, chronic thoughts of suicide, frequent episodes of NSSI), which makes it difficult to discern when a patient is at imminent risk of making a serious suicide attempt. Even with careful attention to suicide risk, it is often difficult to predict serious self-harm or suicide because this behavior can occur impulsively and without warning. Because of the heightened risk of suicide attempts and suicide death in individuals with BPD, it is important that patients be monitored for suicide risk, suicide risk assessments be documented, individualized safety plans be developed (Nuij et al. 2021; Stanley and Brown 2012; Stanley et al. 2018), and treatment plans be adjusted or reformulated as clinically necessary.

APA's *Practice Guidelines for the Psychiatric Evaluation of Adults*, 3rd Edition (American Psychiatric Association 2016a) include detailed information on specific elements to assess in making a determination about suicide risk (see Table 2). Structured approaches to assessing suicide risk can also be helpful for asking about and documenting suicide-related risk information in a consistent fashion. Examples of such approaches include the Suicide Assessment Five-Step Evaluation and Triage for Clinicians (SAFE-T) framework (Substance Abuse and Mental Health Services Administration 2009) and the Assessment of Suicide and Risk Inventory (ASARI; T. Black 2013; Health Standards Organization 2023).

If suicidal ideas, plans, or intent are reported, these should be addressed with the patient. Collaborating with the patient in developing an individualized crisis prevention or safety plan is an essential component of this process (Nuij et al. 2021; Stanley and Brown 2012; Stanley et al. 2018). In the absence of acute factors increasing suicide risk, chronic aspects of risk can typically be addressed in the context of therapy. However, the clinician should also be mindful of situations such as feelings of rejection, fears of abandonment, changes in treating clinicians, or conflicts in interpersonal relationships that may have precipitated suicidal ideas or behaviors in an individual patient in the past. When co-occurring disorders are present that may increase suicide risk (e.g., depressive episodes, AUD or other SUDs), these should be addressed as part of the treatment plan, if not already being treated.

If significant acute suicide risk is present, actions such as hospitalization may be needed to provide more intensive observation and treatment and to reduce the risk of serious self-harm. Referral to a more intensive level of care may also be needed if self-injurious behaviors are frequent. If patients with high levels of suicide risk do not appear to be responding to treatment, consultation with a colleague can be useful.

Risk for Aggressive Behavior

Anger and impulsivity are other aspects of emotional dysregulation that are common in individuals with BPD and can be directed inwardly or at others, including the clinician. Anger is particularly likely to occur when there is a disruption in the patient's relationships or when the patient feels frustrated, abandoned, betrayed, or seriously misunderstood. Thus, it can be helpful to gain a better understanding of the patient's internal experience and its association with anger while emphasizing the need to maintain boundaries of acceptable behavior for purposes of safety. As with suicide risk, it is important for patients to be monitored for risks of aggression, for such risk assessments to be documented, and for treatment plans to be adjusted or reformulated as clinically necessary. However, even with close monitoring and attention to anger, impulsivity, and aggression risk, it is difficult to predict their occurrence. In addition, a complicating factor is that the patient's anger or behavior may produce anger in the therapist, which has the potential to adversely affect clinical judgment.

APA's *Practice Guidelines for the Psychiatric Evaluation of Adults*, 3rd Edition (American Psychiatric Association 2016a) include detailed information on specific elements to assess when determining a patient's risk of aggressive behaviors (see Table 2). In terms of BPD, patients who also have antisocial personality traits or antisocial personality disorder may be at further risk of aggression to others, and severe antisocial features may limit the viability of psychotherapy. Aggression may also be more likely when an SUD is present (Zanarini et al. 2017), when anger is intense (Neukel et al. 2022), when impulsivity and intense anger occur in the presence of identity disturbance (Harford et al. 2019), or when an individual has experienced verbal, emotional, physical, or sexual abuse during adulthood (Zanarini et al. 2017). Contacts with law enforcement or the criminal justice system can occur in individuals with BPD (Epshteyn and Mahmoud 2021; Nakic et al. 2022; Wetterborg et al. 2015) and may be more common in those who experience anger as a prominent symptom (Kolla et al. 2017; McGonigal and Dixon-Gordon 2020). In addition, men with BPD may be more likely to present with externalizing symptoms, such as anger, than women with BPD (Qian et al. 2022).

If the risk of aggression is substantial or if violence appears to be imminent, a higher level of care or hospitalization may be needed to provide more intensive evaluation and observation, to help the patient regain control, and to adjust the treatment plan to reduce risk. Whenever an individual has aggressive or homicidal ideas or behaviors, it is important to identify any intended targets of aggression. If a specific target is identified, the clinician should use clinical judgment to decide whether the patient requires a more supervised setting of care (to provide protection for the identified target and more intensive treatment for the patient), whether the identified target should be warned of the potential for harm, or both. Case law and statutes that address the Tarasoff duty to protect vary considerably by state (Soulier et al. 2010), and clinicians should become familiar with the requirements of their local jurisdiction.

Monitoring and Reassessing the Patient's Clinical Status and Treatment Plan

As treatment proceeds, iterative reevaluation of treatment effectiveness is essential. Although discussions with the patient, family members, and others typically occur as part of the initial assessment (see Statement 1), additional input is helpful as treatment proceeds and the treatment plan is updated. Discussion with parents or other involved caregivers is particularly important when treating adolescents and emerging adults.

Often, the course of treatment is uneven, and setbacks may occur (e.g., at times of heightened stress). Such setbacks do not necessarily indicate that the treatment is ineffective. Rather, therapeutic efforts may facilitate coping strategies to address such situational precipitants. Nonetheless, it is reasonable to expect an overall trend toward improvement.

Features of BPD are heterogeneous. For example, some patients display prominent affective instability, whereas others exhibit marked impulsivity or antisocial traits. Because of this heterogeneity, and because of each patient's unique history, the treatment plan needs to be flexible and adapted to the needs of the individual patient. Flexibility is also needed to respond to the changing characteristics of patients over time (e.g., at one point, the treatment focus may be on safety, whereas at another, it may be on improving relationships and functioning at work). Similarly, the clinician may need to use different treatment modalities or refer the patient for additional treatments (e.g., behavioral, supportive, or psychodynamic psychotherapy) at different times during the treatment or if prior treatments have not been associated with a sufficient clinical response.

If improvement is not occurring or if there are significant changes in presenting issues or symptoms, the diagnosis and treatment plan should be reassessed and a change in the approach to treatment should be considered. When changes to the treatment plan are made, attention should be paid to careful and adequate documentation, including the decision-making process, communication with other clinicians, and the rationale for the treatment change, including aspects related to risk of suicidal or aggressive behaviors. Consultation with a colleague can also be useful when a patient is not improving, for unusually high-risk patients (e.g., when suicide risk is very high), or when it is unclear what the best treatment approach might be. When a consultation has occurred, it is important to document the colleague's recommendations, whether those recommendations were followed or not, and, if the clinician made a different treatment decision, why the recommendations were not followed.

Addressing Co-occurring Psychiatric Disorders

Patients with BPD often have other co-occurring psychiatric disorders, such as mood disorders, PTSD, anxiety disorders, eating disorders, ADHD, SUDs, and other personality disorders (Choi-Kain et al. 2022; Friborg et al. 2014; Geluk Rouwhorst et al. 2023; Grant et al. 2016; Gunderson et al. 2014; Keuroghlian et al. 2015; Leichsenring et al. 2011; Lenzenweger et al. 2007; McDermid et al. 2015; McGlashan et al. 2000; Miller et al. 2022; Momen et al. 2022; Santo et al. 2022; Tate et al. 2022; Trull et al. 2018; Zanarini et al. 2004a, 2010, 2019; Zimmerman et al. 2017). When the presence of co-occurring disorders has been studied in adolescents with BPD, similar increases in the frequency of internalizing and externalizing disorders have been found (Fonagy et al. 2015; Ha et al. 2014; Sharp and Fonagy 2015). These disorders can complicate the clinical picture and need to be addressed in treatment. Furthermore, when a co-occurring disorder is present, the clinical presentation may be more severe, and symptom remission is often more difficult to achieve in the co-occurring disorder (Ceresa et al. 2021; Geluk Rouwhorst et al. 2023; Gunderson et al. 2014; Keuroghlian et al. 2015).

Mood Disorders

BPD is common among patients with bipolar disorder, affecting about one in five bipolar patients overall and an even greater proportion of those with bipolar II disorder (Fornaro et al. 2016). In patients with MDD, estimates suggest that about 15% have BPD (Friborg et al. 2014). Conversely, almost all individuals with BPD will have at least one episode of MDD in their lifetime (Gunderson et al. 2008), and depressive episodes are often recurrent and/or persistent (Gunderson et al. 2008; Skodol et al. 2011).

In patients with BPD, it can be challenging to distinguish mood episodes of bipolar disorder or MDD from mood-related symptoms and affective instability due to BPD. Prior to considering specific treatments for symptoms of depression or affective instability, it is important to establish whether MDD or bipolar disorder is present. This will usually require a detailed longitudinal history of symptoms, treatments, and treatment responses, as well as specific information about associated symptoms and patterns of symptoms, family history of mood disorders, and history from collateral informants. For example, individuals can experience suicidal ideas and hopelessness as elements of depressive episodes or BPD; however, neurovegetative symptoms are more commonly seen with MDD, whereas fears of abandonment, feelings of emptiness, self-destructive behaviors, and NSSI are more consistent with a diagnosis of BPD (American Psychiatric Association 2022a). The presence of psychotic symptoms and a family history of bipolar disorder are also more likely in individuals with bipolar disorder as compared with those who have BPD alone (Durdurak et al. 2022). When compared with individuals with mood disorders alone, individuals with BPD and co-occurring mood disorder are more likely to have atypical features of depression (Gremaud-Heitz et al. 2014), aggressive features (Tong et al. 2021), and suicidal behaviors (Söderholm et al. 2020).

If concomitant bipolar disorder is present in a patient with BPD, there is limited evidence on the optimal approach to treatment (Frankenburg and Zanarini 2002; Gartlehner et al. 2021). Although lamotrigine appears to have efficacy in patients with bipolar depressive episodes (Yildiz et al. 2023), a large randomized controlled trial (RCT) in patients with BPD alone showed no significant clinical effect on BPD (Crawford et al. 2018). Information on treatment with valproic acid or lithium in individuals with bipolar disorder and BPD is even more limited. Lithium treatment is effective in the treatment and prevention of manic episodes (Fountoulakis et al. 2022) and is associated with a decrease in long-term risk of suicide in patients with bipolar disorder in most (Chen et al. 2023; Wilkinson et al. 2023) but not all (Wortzel et al. 2023) studies. Nevertheless, its narrow therapeutic index and toxicity in overdose are important to keep in mind (Barroilhet and Ghaemi 2020; Wortzel et al. 2023) for patients with BPD and bipolar disorder who have significant impulsivity and risk for suicide.

When MDD and BPD co-occur, some data suggest that patients may be less likely to respond to treatments for depression than patients with MDD alone. Nevertheless, many such patients will respond to evidence-based treatments for MDD (Ceresa et al. 2021), and the initial choice of an antidepressant should follow guideline-based recommendations (American Psychiatric Association 2010; Department of Veterans Affairs/Department of Defense 2022). In addition, treatment of BPD may improve the chance of depression response (Ceresa et al. 2021). Several small studies of selective serotonin reuptake inhibitors (SSRIs) showed benefits in patients with MDD and BPD (Ceresa et al. 2021). Because of their frequent use in the treatment of MDD alone, SSRIs tend to be used most often in patients with co-occurring MDD and BPD (Ceresa et al. 2021; Pascual et al. 2023). Serotonin-norepinephrine reuptake inhibitors (SNRIs) have not been well studied in patients with BPD and MDD. Several small studies in the older literature suggested that monoamine oxidase inhibitors (MAOIs) may be more beneficial than tricyclic antidepressants (TCAs) in individuals with BPD (Cowdry and Gardner 1988; Parsons et al. 1989), particularly if atypical depressive symptoms are present. Although MAOIs can be an option in individuals with MDD whose depressive symptoms have not responded to other antidepressive treatments (Van den Eynde et al. 2022a), they are rarely used in patients with MDD and BPD. If considered, factors such as impulsivity, concomitant substance use, and suicidal behaviors should be weighed carefully because of the potential for drug-drug and drug-diet interactions (Van den Eynde et al. 2022a, 2022b) with MAOI treatment.

Because patients with BPD can have significant suicide risk and repeated suicidal attempts or hospitalizations for suicidal ideation, they are sometimes referred for ECT on this basis. As noted earlier, before considering treatment such as ECT, it is important to establish whether mood-related symptoms, including suicide-related risks, are related to a concomitant mood disorder rather than attributable to BPD. As with other antidepressant treatments in individuals with BPD, most of the available evidence suggests that patients with concomitant BPD and mood disorder can respond to ECT (Feske et al. 2004; Hein et al. 2022a, 2022b; Kaster et al. 2018; Rasmussen 2015). Despite this, when BPD and MDD co-occur, response to ECT may be slower, remission and response rates may be less robust, and relapse may be more frequent after ECT treatment is stopped than in depressed patients without BPD (Feske et al. 2004; Hein et al. 2022a, 2022b; Kaster et al. 2018; Rasmussen 2015). These factors should be weighed along with the other potential benefits and risks of ECT before making specific treatment recommendations. Although data on benefits of TMS are more limited than data on ECT in patients with concomitant MDD and BPD, there is less potential risk, particularly in terms of cognitive side effects (Cailhol et al. 2014; Chiappini et al. 2022; Feffer et al. 2022; Konstantinou et al. 2021; Reyes-López et al. 2018). In addition, one study suggested that response to TMS in patients with BPD is comparable with that in patients without BPD (Ward et al. 2021).

Even less is known about the use of ketamine to treat depressive episodes in patients with BPD who have co-occurring bipolar disorder or MDD. In patients with BPD, a small RCT of a single infusion of ketamine, as compared with midazolam, showed no effects on the primary outcome of suicidal ideation or secondary outcomes of anxiety, depression, or BPD symptoms, although socio-occupational functioning was better with ketamine at 14 days (Fineberg et al. 2023). In terms of potential adverse effects, one case report suggested that intravenous ketamine might be associated with worsening symptoms of BPD (Vanicek et al. 2022). The occurrence of dissociative symptoms in other studies of ketamine treatment (Fineberg et al. 2023; McIntyre et al. 2021; Rhee et al. 2022; Williamson et al. 2023) also suggests that caution and careful monitoring should be used if ketamine is prescribed to treat depressive episodes in an individual with BPD.

Anxiety Disorders

Anxiety disorders, like mood disorders, are common in individuals with BPD (Ansell et al. 2011; Leichsenring et al. 2023; McGlashan et al. 2000; Qadeer Shah et al. 2023; Zanarini et al. 1998, 2004a; Zimmerman and Mattia 1999) and may represent an initial reason for patient assessment (Zimmerman and Becker 2023). Reported rates of anxiety disorders vary with the sampling method and setting of care in clinical samples; however, rates of panic disorder and social phobia are high in individuals with BPD, occurring in one-fifth to almost one-half of some samples (McGlashan et al. 2000; Qadeer Shah et al. 2023; Zanarini et al. 1998, 2004a; Zimmerman and Mattia 1999). Simple phobias are reported in about one-quarter of individuals with BPD, whereas generalized anxiety disorder and obsessive-compulsive disorder (OCD) occur in one-sixth to one-fifth of the samples (McGlashan et al. 2000; Qadeer Shah et al. 2023; Zanarini et al. 1998, 2004a; Zimmerman and Mattia 1999). Information on the course of co-occurring anxiety disorders in BPD is limited because many of the available studies enrolled inpatients. Nevertheless, when assessed longitudinally, the prevalence of anxiety disorders in patients with BPD appears to fluctuate as symptoms remit and recur and as some individuals develop a new anxiety disorder diagnosis (Silverman et al. 2012; Zanarini et al. 2004a). In addition, the overall proportion of anxiety diagnoses appears to decrease somewhat with time, although it remains elevated relative to individuals with other personality disorders (Silverman et al. 2012; Zanarini et al. 2004a) or rates of anxiety disorders in general community samples (Kessler et al. 1994).

In terms of anxiety disorder treatment, few studies have assessed specific treatment approaches in patients with co-occurring BPD (Harned and Valenstein 2013; Pascual et al. 2023). Consequently, treatment approaches typically include the addition of anxiety-focused elements to psychotherapy or the use of antidepressants, if appropriate, for treatment of the co-occurring anxiety disorder. Use of benzodiazepines is not generally recommended because of the potential for greater impulsivity or disinhibition, as well as the potential for misuse or the development of dependence (Leichsenring et al. 2023; Lieslehto et al. 2023; Pascual et al. 2023).

Eating Disorders

The co-occurrence of BPD and eating disorders varies with the specific eating disorder and its subtype. Rates of BPD are greatest among individuals with bulimia nervosa and the binge-purge subtype of anorexia nervosa as compared with the restrictive subtype (Reas et al. 2013; Sansone et al. 2005; Skodol et al. 1993).

Among clinical samples of patients with BPD, eating disorder diagnoses were frequent, with greater rates among inpatient than outpatient samples (Chen et al. 2009; Martinussen et al. 2017; Zanarini et al. 2021). Symptoms related to eating are also common in patients with BPD even when full criteria for an eating disorder are not met (Marino and Zanarini 2001). Notably, most studies on BPD and eating disorder co-occurrence have been done in women with either anorexia nervosa or bulimia nervosa; limited information is available on individuals of other genders or those with binge-eating disorder.

As in BPD, in adults, the primary treatment for anorexia nervosa or for binge-eating disorder is an evidence-based psychotherapy, either alone or in combination with an SSRI (e.g., fluoxetine) recommended for bulimia nervosa (American Psychiatric Association 2023). In adolescents and emerging adults who have an involved caregiver, an eating disorder–focused family-based treatment is recommended for treatment of anorexia nervosa and suggested for that of bulimia nervosa (American Psychiatric Association 2023). Consequently, for individuals with a co-occurring diagnosis of BPD and an eating disorder, psychotherapy may be able to address both conditions simultaneously. In other circumstances, with medical instability or significant nutritional compromise, stabilization of the eating disorder may be needed (American Psychiatric Association 2023) prior to initiating treatment for BPD.

Substance Use Disorders

SUDs, including AUD, are also common in patients with BPD (Carpenter et al. 2016; Grant et al. 2016; Santo et al. 2022; Trull et al. 2018). Patients with BPD and co-occurring SUDs often have poorer outcomes than those with BPD alone, and the risks are greater for morbidity and mortality related to injuries or suicidal behaviors (Doyle et al. 2016; Heath et al. 2018a; Kjær et al. 2020). Substance use may heighten risks of being victimized (Seid et al. 2022; Victor and Hedden-Clayton 2023) and can also increase impulsivity and lower the threshold for acting on self-injurious behaviors. Consequently, inquiring about substance use is an important aspect of history taking. It is also helpful to provide patients with education on the risks of substance use in the context of BPD. When substance use is present, motivational interviewing and brief interventions can be used as initial steps. For individuals with an SUD, concomitant treatment or referral for treatment is essential. Depending on the severity of the SUD, stabilization may be needed before initiating BPD treatment, and inpatient treatment may be needed for withdrawal management or more intensive interventions. For some patients, participation in a community-based peer support group such as a 12-step program can be helpful, although there is a paucity of research on these modalities (Ferri et al. 2006). Nevertheless, the focus and structure of groups can vary considerably, and, in some instances, emotional distress or harm can occur in relation to issues such as boundary management. For these reasons, community-based peer support programs cannot substitute for formal medical treatment in the management of SUDs.

Evidence-based pharmacotherapy (e.g., opioid agonist or antagonist treatment for opioid use disorder, acamprosate or naltrexone for AUD) should also be recommended when appropriate to the patient's clinical condition. In addition to the benefits of oral and LAI naltrexone in AUD (Bahji et al. 2022; Kedia et al. 2023; Murphy et al. 2022), oral naltrexone has been noted to reduce self-injurious behavior in open-label studies (Roth et al. 1996), retrospective analyses (Timäus et al. 2021), and case reports (Griengl et al. 2001; McGee 1997). However, clinical observations suggest that, in some patients treated with naltrexone, self-injurious behavior may escalate in frequency or severity rather than decline. If patients are receiving medication treatment through an SUD treatment program or primary care clinician, ongoing communication and coordination of care is important as described earlier in the section "Coordinating the Treatment Effort."

Posttraumatic Stress Disorder

In comparison with the general population or comparison groups with other psychiatric disorders, individuals with BPD have higher rates of having experienced childhood adversity or traumatic experiences as an adult (de Aquino Ferreira et al. 2018; Hailes et al. 2019; Porter et al. 2020; Solmi et al. 2021). Individuals may also have experienced trauma related to discrimination, such as that related to race, ethnicity, sexual orientation, or sex/gender (Maharaj et al. 2021; Spengler et al. 2016; Sue et al. 2007). Among individuals with BPD, there is an increased incidence of PTSD (Scheiderer et al. 2015) and concomitant symptoms of PTSD can occur without meeting full criteria for a diagnosis of PTSD (American Psychiatric Association 2022a). Notably, individuals with both disorders have greater rates of exposure to multiple and interpersonal trauma than individuals with either disorder alone (Jowett et al. 2020a). Although there can be some overlap of BPD with the features of complex PTSD, these two conditions appear to be conceptually and clinically distinct (Ford and Courtois 2021; Giourou et al. 2018; Jowett et al. 2020b; Maercker et al. 2022).

In terms of treatment for PTSD, individuals who have concomitant BPD typically require a phased approach to treatment in which exposure-based treatment is begun only after solidifying the therapeutic alliance and stabilizing BPD symptoms, including significant suicide risk. Although meta-analyses have not shown an increase in adverse effects when exposure-based treatments are used to treat PTSD in patients with BPD, the available studies have typically used a phased approach and excluded patients with significant suicide risk (Slotema et al. 2020; Zeifman et al. 2021). DBT has been used to treat PTSD; results of one RCT showed benefit with DBT as compared with a wait-list control group (Bohus et al. 2013). Notably, in the subgroup of patients with co-occurring PTSD and BPD, the reduction in PTSD symptoms was comparable with that seen in patients with PTSD only (Bohus et al. 2013), whereas BPD symptoms were less responsive to DBT when PTSD was present as compared with BPD alone (Barnicot and Priebe 2013). In comparative effectiveness studies in patients with PTSD, comparable outcomes were found with DBT and cognitive processing therapy (CPT) (Bohus et al. 2020). Another comparison of DBT and GPM for PTSD showed that both treatments were associated with comparable improvement in PTSD symptoms, but patients with co-occurring PTSD began and ended with more symptoms than those with BPD alone (Boritz et al. 2016).

Eye movement desensitization and reprocessing (EMDR) is another treatment approach that has been studied in PTSD (Cuijpers et al. 2020; Hudays et al. 2022; Mavranezouli et al. 2020) and suggested or recommended as a PTSD treatment in several practice guidelines (Courtois et al. 2017; Department of Veterans Affairs/Department of Defense 2023; Martin et al. 2021). Most research suggests that the effects of EMDR are comparable with those of CBT; however, many of these studies have significant biases. When meta-analyses have focused on studies with a low risk of bias, benefits of EMDR appear less robust (Cuijpers et al. 2020; Hudays et al. 2022; Mavranezouli et al. 2020). In patients with BPD and PTSD, only pilot data are available, which is insufficient to support EMDR use in this context (Wilhelmus et al. 2023).

Some individuals with BPD may experience auditory hallucinations, dissociative symptoms, or both; each of these symptoms may be more common in individuals with BPD who have experienced trauma. When auditory hallucinations are present, they are often related to stress. In contrast to hallucinations in schizophrenia, individuals with BPD who experience hallucinations will not typically have formal thought disorder, flat or blunted affect, or negative symptoms (Beatson et al. 2019; Niemantsverdriet et al. 2017; Slotema et al. 2018). Although psychotic symptoms are mild and transient in most patients with BPD, the presence of more severe or persistent psychosis should prompt additional evaluation for a concomitant psychotic disorder such as schizophrenia.

Dissociative symptoms, including depersonalization and derealization, can be transient but can also be severe or frequent and interfere with treatment and with psychosocial functioning (Bohus et al. 2021; Krause-Utz 2022; Shah et al. 2020). Dissociative identity disorder can also co-occur with BPD (Al-Shamali et al. 2022; Brand and Lanius 2014; Scalabrini et al. 2017). In a transdiagnostic sample, dissociative symptoms were associated with an increased risk of self-harm and suicide attempts (Sommer et al. 2021), whereas in studies of DBT, more severe dissociative symptoms were associated with poorer treatment outcomes (Kleindienst et al. 2011).

Autism Spectrum Disorder

Information on individuals with autism spectrum disorder (ASD) and BPD is limited. Current evidence does not suggest that rates of BPD are increased in individuals with ASD or that rates of ASD are increased in individuals with BPD. However, there has been increasing recognition that distinguishing between BPD and ASD can be difficult because symptoms such as emotional dysregulation, relationship disruptions, and self-injurious behavior can occur in either diagnosis (Cheney et al. 2023; May et al. 2021). In addition, when both disorders are present, features of ASD can make it more difficult for patients to engage in psychotherapy for BPD (Cheney et al. 2023; May et al. 2021).

Treating Patients During Pregnancy and the Postpartum Period

Individuals with childbearing potential and who may become pregnant should be assisted in obtaining effective contraception if pregnancy is not desired. For patients who are planning to become pregnant, are pregnant, or are in the postpartum period, collaborative discussion of treatment options is essential. In addition to the patient, such discussions typically include the obstetrician-gynecologist or other obstetrical practitioner, the infant's pediatrician for individuals who are breastfeeding, and, if involved, a partner or other people in the patient's support network. The overall goal is to develop a plan of care aimed at optimizing outcomes for both the patient and the infant. Untreated or inadequately treated maternal psychiatric illness can result in poor adherence to prenatal care, inadequate nutrition, increased alcohol or tobacco use, and disruptions to the family environment and mother-infant bonding (ACOG Committee on Practice Bulletins—Obstetrics 2008; American Academy of Pediatrics and the American College of Obstetrician-Gynecologists 2017; Tosato et al. 2017). In addition, during pregnancy and the postpartum period, frequent reassessment will be needed to determine if any modifications to the treatment plan are indicated. As with all individuals who are pregnant, regular prenatal care is essential to ensuring optimal outcomes (American Academy of Pediatrics and the American College of Obstetrician-Gynecologists 2017; American College of Obstetricians and Gynecologists 2018).

In patients with BPD, psychotherapy is the primary focus of treatment, and it may be possible to avoid the use of or to discontinue medications prior to conception, during pregnancy, or while breastfeeding. All psychotropic medications studied to date cross the placenta, are present in amniotic fluid, and enter human breast milk (American Academy of Pediatrics and the American College of Obstetrician-Gynecologists 2017). If an individual becomes pregnant while taking a psychotropic medication, consideration should be given to consulting an obstetrician-gynecologist or maternal/fetal medicine subspecialist in addition to discussion with the prescribing clinician to determine whether the risks of stopping the medication outweigh any possible fetal risks (American Academy of Pediatrics and the American College of Obstetrician-Gynecologists 2017; U.S. Food and Drug Administration 2011). For many patients, the period of greatest teratogenic risk (i.e., through the eighth week of gestation) will already have passed before prenatal care begins, and stopping psychotropic medication will not avoid or reduce teratogenic risk (American Academy of Pediatrics and the American College of Obstetrician-Gynecologists 2017). If medications are continued during pregnancy, physiological alterations of pregnancy affect the absorption, distribution, metabolism, and elimination of medications, and adjustments in medication dosages may be needed (ACOG Committee on Practice Bulletins—Obstetrics 2008; Chisolm and Payne 2016).

Individuals who are taking medications and who wish to breastfeed their infants should review the potential benefits of breastfeeding as well as potential risks in the context of shared decision-making (American College of Obstetricians and Gynecologists' Committee on Obstetric Practice and Breastfeeding Expert Work Group 2016; Sachs and Committee On Drugs 2013), with associated monitoring of growth and development by the infant's pediatrician (Sachs and Committee On Drugs 2013).

Addressing Needs of Patients in Correctional Settings

Rates of psychiatric illness, including BPD, are higher in correctional settings (e.g., prisons, jails, police lockups, detention facilities) than in the general population (Al-Rousan et al. 2017; Bebbington et al. 2017; Black et al. 2007; Nakic et al. 2022; Steadman et al. 2009; Wetterborg et al. 2015). Among individuals with BPD, criminal justice involvement may be especially likely in those with concomitant SUDs or antisocial personality disorder (Howard et al. 2021; Mir et al. 2015). Careful assessment and treatment planning are essential when individuals with a psychiatric condition are in correctional settings. Although some aspects of treatment may need to be adjusted to conform with unique aspects of correctional settings (Tamburello et al. 2018), many individuals experience gaps in care during incarceration (Epshteyn and Mahmoud 2021; Fries et al. 2013; Reingle Gonzalez and Connell 2014; Wilper et al. 2009). Access to treatment should be preserved, including treatment for concomitant SUDs (American Psychiatric Association 2007). Suicidal behavior and NSSI are particular risks in the correctional system (Barker et al. 2014; Casiano et al. 2013; Young et al. 2006). In this regard, patients with BPD may also ingest objects or insert them into their body while incarcerated (Frei-Lanter et al. 2012; Mannarino et al. 2017; Masood 2021; Rada and James 1982; Reisner et al. 2013).

While in the correctional system, individuals with BPD may engage in disruptive behavior that results in disciplinary infractions (Yasmeen et al. 2022) and/or placement in a locked-down segregated setting in which inmates typically spend an average of 23 hours/day in a cell, have limited human interaction, and have minimal or no access to programs (American Psychiatric Association 2017, 2018; American Public Health Association 2013; National Commission on Correctional Health Care 2016; Semenza and Grosholz 2019). Such settings offer little support or access to treatment due to security concerns and are likely to exacerbate rather than reduce disruptive behaviors (American College of Correctional Physicians 2013; American Psychiatric Association 2016b, 2017; American Public Health Association 2013; National Commission on Correctional Health Care 2016). Notably, rates of self-injury and suicide appear to be higher in such settings than elsewhere in the correctional system (Baillargeon et al. 2009b; Favril et al. 2020; Glowa-Kollisch et al. 2016; Kaba et al. 2014; Way et al. 2005), which is of particular concern in patients with BPD. Group treatment with Systems Training for Emotional Predictability and Problem Solving (STEPPS) has been studied in a correctional population and is associated with reductions in suicidal behaviors and disciplinary infractions, although attrition rates were significant (Black et al. 2013, 2018).

Continuity of care is also important upon release from a correctional setting. This is particularly true for individuals who have been incarcerated for significant periods of time who will likely need assistance with domains such as housing, treatment needs, and financial support, including Medicaid benefits (American Psychiatric Association 2009; Baillargeon et al. 2009a, 2010; Draine et al. 2010; Wenzlow et al. 2011).

Statement 4 – Discussion of Diagnosis and Treatment

APA *recommends* **(1C)** that a patient with borderline personality disorder be engaged in a collaborative discussion about their diagnosis and treatment, which includes psychoeducation related to the disorder.

Implementation

Once a diagnosis of BPD has been established, it is important to discuss the diagnosis with the patient in a collaborative fashion that allows them to ask questions and share their experiences and perspectives. When treating an adolescent, parents or other involved caregivers should also be engaged in the discussion of the diagnostic impression. Clinicians are sometimes reluctant to document a diagnosis of BPD or to share the diagnosis with patients out of concern for upsetting the patient, disrupting the therapeutic relationship, or contributing to discrimination toward the patient because of stigma against individuals with BPD or those with psychiatric conditions more generally (Lequesne and Hersh 2004; Proctor et al. 2021; Sims et al. 2022; Sisti et al. 2016; Sulzer et al. 2016). However, disclosure and discussion of a BPD diagnosis is preferred by patients (Proctor et al. 2021; Sulzer et al. 2016), does not adversely affect patient satisfaction (Zimmerman et al. 2018), is crucial on ethical grounds (American Medical Association Code of Medical Ethics 2023b), and is part of good clinical practice. In addition, with the passing of the 21st Century Cures Act (Office of the National Coordinator for Health Information Technology 2020), clinical notes are required to be shared with patients except under very limited circumstances, and proactively disclosing and discussing the diagnosis of BPD will aid patients in understanding these notes. For many patients, having access to notes and understanding the information that they contain fosters greater engagement in their own care (DesRoches et al. 2020).

Disclosing a diagnosis of BPD is also an initial step in discussing treatment options as well as in providing psychoeducation about BPD to patients. When psychoeducation is provided in a compassionate, nonjudgmental fashion, it can provide context and validation for the patient's experiences (e.g., in relationships, sense of self, emotional response). It is also important to ask about and understand the patient's beliefs about BPD and its features because patients may have internalized stigma or received misinformation related to the diagnosis (Koivisto et al. 2022; Masland et al. 2023). Typically, topics reviewed as part of psychoeducation include symptoms and behaviors that are often a part of the disorder and the expected types and courses of treatment (American Psychiatric Association 2016a). For patients with BPD, it is particularly important to emphasize that treatment is effective (Ng et al. 2016, 2019a, 2019b). Many patients with BPD benefit from ongoing education about self-care (e.g., safe sex, potential legal problems, balanced diet) as well as education about crisis or safety plans. For patients who also have other concomitant disorders, these can be discussed in terms of their features and treatments in the context of BPD. In addition to psychoeducation provided by the clinician, it can be helpful to share criteria from DSM-5-TR (American Psychiatric Association 2022a), internet resources (Emotions Matter 2023a; Gunderson and Berkowitz 1991; National Education Alliance for Borderline Personality Disorder 2023c; National Institute of Mental Health 2023; New York Presbyterian Hospital 2023), or books on personality traits (Oldham and Morris 1995) or BPD (National Education Alliance for Borderline Personality Disorder 2023a) written for laypersons. More extensive psychoeducational intervention, consisting of workshops, lectures, seminars, or web-based programs may also be helpful.

Family members and other caregivers will often be a key part of the patient's support network and care team, and this is particularly true when treating an adolescent. For this reason, family members and others in the support network will often benefit from receiving educational materials about BPD or being directed to organizations that offer education and support (Emotions Matter 2023a; Mental Health America 2023; National Alliance on Mental Illness 2023; National Education Alliance for Borderline Personality Disorder 2023b; New York Presbyterian Hospital 2023). In addition to providing emotional support, such individuals may also be providing material support such as housing, financial assistance, insurance, transportation, childcare, or other assistance. They may be able to share observations about the patient's symptoms or behaviors, help the patient develop a safety plan, provide opinions about specific treatment approaches, or identify practical barriers to the patient's ability to participate in treatment, such as limitations on insight, geographical issues, lack of transportation, childcare or caregiving responsibilities, financial or insurance coverage constraints, insufficient access to recommended treatment, or other systemic barriers to care. Psychoeducation for families should be distinguished from family therapy, which is sometimes a desirable part of the treatment plan and sometimes not, depending on the patient's history and status of current relationships.

Psychosocial Interventions

Statement 5 – Psychotherapy

APA *recommends* **(1B)** that a patient with borderline personality disorder be treated with a structured approach to psychotherapy that has support in the literature and targets the core features of the disorder.

Implementation

Psychotherapy is at the core of treatment for BPD for adolescents and adults. A structured approach that has support in the literature is recommended. The specific psychotherapeutic approach selected should target the core features of the disorder.

With all psychotherapeutic modalities, it is important to foster a positive, trusting therapeutic alliance, convey a validating and nonjudgmental attitude, and balance active support with an impetus to change and develop self-efficacy. Setting a framework for treatment is also crucial (see the "Implementation" section for Statement 3), although aspects of the therapeutic framework will depend on the type of structured psychotherapy for BPD being used. Teaching of skills and development of crisis plans are elements of treatment that are shared by many psychotherapies for BPD, whereas other psychotherapies have a basis in psychodynamic principles and focus on helping patients use the therapeutic relationship to address problematic defensive patterns and understand their own and others' mental states (Bohus et al. 2021; Leichsenring et al. 2023). In adolescents and young adults, psychotherapy will typically need to address developmental issues (Sharp and Wall 2018) and to incorporate family members or other caregivers as part of psychotherapy. For adults, family members and others in the patient's support network may also be involved in treatment. Developmental tasks may also warrant exploration at other points in the individual's life.

Multiple structured approaches to psychotherapy are available and have been studied in patients with BPD (see Appendix C, Statement 5, and Appendix D); characteristics of these approaches are summarized in Table 3. Structured psychotherapies for BPD have an associated manual or protocol and typically incorporate ongoing supervision. These factors build on initial training and supervision in the use of a specific psychotherapy and help support delivery of treatment with a high degree of fidelity.

Although a number of structured approaches to psychotherapy that target BPD are superior to treatment-as-usual or wait-list control conditions, there is no clear evidence that any specific struc-

TABLE 3. Comparison of characteristics of psychotherapies for borderline personality disorder (BPD)

Characteristic	Dialectical behavior therapy (DBT)	Dynamic deconstructive psychotherapy (DDP)	Mentalization-based treatment (MBT)	Schema-focused therapy (SFT)	Systems Training for Emotional Predictability and Problem Solving (STEPPS)	Transference-focused psychotherapy (TFP)	Good psychiatric management (GPM)
Typical treatment duration	6–12 months	12–18 months	12–18 months	Depends on format	20 weeks	12–18 months	12 months
Individual therapy	1 hour/week	1 hour/week	1 hour/week	2 hours/week for 3 years	Not part of treatment	Two 45- to 50-minute sessions/week	Once weekly as needed
Group therapy	1.5 hour/week	Not part of treatment	75–90 minutes/week	90 minutes/week for 8 months	2 hours/week	Used as indicated	Encouraged
Family therapy/involvement	Multifamily group for adolescents Family groups for adults	Not part of the treatment	MBT-Family MBT-Family Group Therapy	Not part of treatment	1 hour session	Used as indicated	Family psychoeducation
Crisis management	Minimize emergency department (ED) use Focus on use of skills and skills coaching Between-session availability	Exploration in session	On-call mentalizing team or ED after hours	Individualized plans	Use skills in group with referral to ED or individual therapist, as needed	Minimize ED use, and use only when absolutely necessary	Crisis plan or algorithm regarding inter-session contact
Manual available for treatment in adolescents	Yes	No	Yes	No	No	Yes	Yes
Comments	DBT skills training can be used independently from other DBT components			Delivered in an individual or group format but not both	Supplements other treatment		

tured approaches to psychotherapy of BPD have significantly superior outcomes to other BPD-focused structured psychotherapeutic modalities in either adults or adolescents (Storebø et al. 2020; see Statement 5 in Appendix C). In addition, limited information is available on treatment of men, gender minorities, or non-White individuals or those with Hispanic ethnicity (Storebø et al. 2020; see Statement 5 in Appendix C). In most studies that compare two active treatments, both types of psychotherapy are associated with clinical improvement, even when the outcomes of the therapies do not differ with respect to one another (see Appendices C and D). As such, selection of a treatment approach will depend on factors such as patient preferences for treatment, the availability of specific treatments, and the resource requirements of a treatment (Bohus et al. 2021; Choi-Kain et al. 2016, 2017). Under some circumstances, a patient may be unable or prefer not to access a structured form of psychotherapy for BPD (e.g., due to availability, insurance coverage, affordability of a specific psychotherapy, other reasons related to logistics or patient preference). In this situation, less structured supportive psychotherapy may still produce clinical improvements via ongoing treatment engagement, including building a therapeutic alliance and providing psychoeducation (see Statement 3).

In terms of the optimal duration of psychotherapy for BPD, evidence is also limited in terms of the time needed to resolve interpersonal problems and to attain and maintain lasting improvements in personality-related dysfunction and overall functioning. Most studies of structured psychotherapies for BPD have ranged in duration from 6 months to 18 months (Storebø et al. 2020; see Appendix D). In one longitudinal study, a majority of patients continued in some form of outpatient treatment for much of a 6-year period of follow-up (Zanarini et al. 2004b). Although other treatment trials have been of shorter duration, study participants often continue to receive other treatment, including psychotherapy for BPD, after completion of the research trials. In addition, a significant number of patients with BPD do not fully respond to initial treatment (Woodbridge et al. 2022) and may require longer periods of treatment. It is also unclear whether the optimal treatment duration varies with specific BPD features, overall severity, or with treatment intensity. For example, in an inpatient sample of individuals with BPD, many with co-occurring disorders, an intensive multimodal therapeutic approach that incorporated a mentalization-based therapeutic model was associated with a significant degree of benefit on multiple outcomes with an average length of stay of 6 weeks (Fowler et al. 2018).

DBT is a multicomponent approach that has efficacy in treating adolescents and adults with BPD but may also be useful in treating patients with other diagnoses who are at significant risk for suicide (Linehan 1993a, 1993b; Linehan et al. 2015). A key focus of DBT is to help patients develop a proactive problem-solving approach and to learn to tolerate stress, regulate emotions, improve interpersonal effectiveness, and develop mindfulness (i.e., an ability to focus awareness on the present moment) as a way to address emotional dysregulation. At the core of the therapy is a philosophical dialectic between self-acceptance and strategies aimed at change. Skills worksheets and a specific protocol for addressing suicidal thoughts and behaviors are incorporated in the therapy. DBT is administered by a team of clinicians and is time intensive for clinical teams as well as for patients. It typically includes 6–12 months of treatment with 1 hour of individual therapy and 90 minutes of group skills training weekly. Treatment team members are also available by cellphone for skills coaching between sessions. Weekly therapist consultation is an integral part of the treatment.

DBT skills training has also been studied as a standalone treatment and showed comparable effects to the full multicomponent approach to DBT when individual therapy was replaced with a case management intervention (Linehan et al. 2015). As a less intensive intervention, DBT skills training may be more accessible than multicomponent DBT. Manual-assisted CBT, a 10-session intervention, can also be considered as a less intensive approach in the treatment of individuals with BPD (Davidson et al. 2014; Tyrer et al. 2004; Weinberg et al. 2006).

As the name implies, MBT focuses on mentalization, the ability to reflect on one's thoughts and feelings as well as those of others. Without such an ability, it is challenging to have a realistic emotional perspective on interpersonal events, particularly under stress. In MBT, the therapist guides the patient in learning to assess the emotional aspects of stressful interpersonal situations, such as those related to attachment, and then adopt a more realistic behavioral response (Bateman and Fonagy 2004, 2009; Jørgensen et al. 2013). The therapeutic relationship can also provide examples for working through these steps, although transference interpretations are not used. MBT typically includes 12–18 months of treatment with 50 minutes of weekly individual therapy and 75–90 minutes of group therapy. In adolescents, family therapy is incorporated in the treatment instead of group therapy. A weekly team meeting is also part of the treatment protocol.

TFP is a manualized, psychodynamically oriented psychotherapy that uses the transference relationship to help address intense emotional states and difficulties in interpersonal relationships (Caligor et al. 2018; Clarkin et al. 2007; Doering et al. 2010; Giesen-Bloo et al. 2006; Yeomans et al. 2015). A core principle of TFP is the belief that internal images of the self in relation to others, based on developmental experiences, exist in the mind of all people. These mental images of self in relation to others are connected by strong emotions. In BPD, the internal mental images are extreme, intense, and polarized due to biological and developmental influences. *Transference* is the activation of these internal images in interactions with people. In the structured setting of therapy, this activation of the internal images of the self in relation to others can be observed and understood as they are experienced in relation to the therapist. This treatment model engages reflection on the emotions being experienced in the moment, along with reflection on the reasons that the images are extreme and polarized. This joint reflection on internal states helps the patient to modulate affects better and to experience both the self and relations with others in a more complex and realistic way. TFP typically includes 12–18 months of individual therapy delivered for 50 minutes twice weekly. TFP concepts and techniques can also be incorporated into other settings (Hersh et al. 2017). Supervision is recommended for clinicians who treat patients with TFP.

DDP is a manualized individual psychotherapy (Gregory 2022; Gregory and Remen 2008), derived from psychodynamic psychotherapy, that uses the philosophical concept of deconstruction as a framework for treatment. Links to neurobiology and object relations are also part of the theoretical foundation of DDP. Therapeutic interventions focus on approaches such as alliance building, reflective listening, describing affect-laden experiences as simple narratives, recognizing and addressing polarized attributions, learning to assess oneself from an external perspective, and facilitating mourning of the limitations of oneself and others (Gregory 2022). Recent interpersonal experiences serve as primary examples for discussion, although dream exploration, artwork, or creative writing can also be used. DDP typically includes 12–18 months of treatment delivered weekly in 45- to 50-minute sessions. Other interventions such as interpersonally focused group therapy, art therapy, or 12-step programs can supplement DDP.

SFT is based on the concept that individuals view themselves and others in terms of cognitive "schemas" that are an outgrowth of developmental experiences and that manifest themselves in persistent patterns of thinking, feeling, and behaving, although they are often outside of conscious awareness (Arntz and van Genderen 2021; Farrell et al. 2009; Giesen-Bloo et al. 2006; Young et al. 2003). In BPD, dysfunctional "schema modes" are seen as strongly held and controlling a person's life through recurring and rapidly shifting constellations of intense emotions, thoughts, feelings, and behaviors. These dysfunctional schema modes are addressed by fostering attachment between the patient and therapist as well as by applying behavioral, cognitive, and experiential techniques (including homework assignments). SFT also incorporates emotional awareness training and psychoeducation and employs individualized plans for managing distress. In clinical trials, SFT has been delivered in individual 50-minute twice weekly sessions for 3 years (Giesen-Bloo et al. 2006) or in weekly 90-minute group sessions for 8 months (Farrell et al. 2009).

STEPPS is designed as a supplement to other treatment approaches and is delivered in a seminar format using detailed lesson plans (Bartels and Crotty 1992; Blum et al. 2008; STEPPS 2022). STEPPS consists of weekly 2-hour groups for 20 weeks as well as a single 2-hour session for families. It incorporates psychoeducation and skills training in emotional and behavioral management, viewed from the context of social and family systems. Participants are asked to monitor their thoughts, feelings, and behaviors over the course of the program to increase their awareness and identify improvements.

GPM uses a multimodal case management model in which BPD is understood as a reflection of interpersonal hypersensitivity (Gunderson et al. 2018; Links 2014; McMain et al. 2009). As originally studied (McMain et al. 2009), GPM was developed using psychodynamic principles. Treatment uses a generalist model that emphasizes improvements in vocational and social functioning and incorporates psychoeducation about BPD, as well as psychopharmacological management when clinically appropriate (Gunderson et al. 2018; Links 2014). The therapy uses a here-and-now approach in which the therapist shows interest in the patient's experiences and the interpersonal context and thoughts that precede their feelings and behaviors. It also focuses on the therapeutic alliance, including attention to signs that a negative transference may be developing. GPM is typically delivered in once-weekly sessions with weekly therapist supervision. An advantage of GPM is that it is relatively easy for clinicians to learn and apply (Bernanke and McCommon 2018; Hong 2016; Links et al. 2015). It has also been adapted for use with adolescents (Ilagan and Choi-Kain 2021). In addition, training in GPM may improve clinician attitudes about treating patients with BPD (Keuroghlian et al. 2016; Klein et al. 2022b; Masland et al. 2018).

Pharmacotherapy

Statement 6 – Clinical Review Before Medication Initiation

APA *recommends* **(1C)** that a patient with borderline personality disorder have a review of co-occurring disorders, prior psychotherapies, other nonpharmacological treatments, past medication trials, and current medications before initiating any new medication.

Implementation

Psychotherapy is the primary modality recommended for use in the treatment of BPD. As such, it is important to learn about a patient's past and current psychotherapies, including the types, the clinician's fidelity to treatment principles, the treatment intensity and duration, and the patient's experience with therapy if this information was not already obtained as part of the initial evaluations (see Statement 1). Such information is helpful in determining whether a current psychotherapy can be optimized before adding medication or whether a change in the psychotherapeutic approach may be needed.

Similarly, it is important to obtain information about prior medication trials, including the dosages, durations, effectiveness, and associated adverse effects if this information was not already obtained as part of the initial evaluations (see Statement 1). A review of current medications is also important to determine whether the patient has been able to obtain, adhere to, and tolerate the medication. If the medication has been ineffective or if the response has been insufficient, it may be possible to increase the dosage of the medication in an effort to achieve therapeutic benefit. Alternatively, if response has been minimal, it may be preferable to discontinue the medication and reassess the need for pharmacotherapy.

Half or more of BPD patients receive polypharmacy (Bridler et al. 2015; Gartlehner et al. 2021; Paris 2015; Romanowicz et al. 2020; Shapiro-Thompson and Fineberg 2022; Soler et al. 2022; Starcevic and Janca 2018), and drug-drug interactions may affect efficacy and tolerability by increasing or decreasing serum medication levels. Consequently, the medication regimen should be examined as a whole, rather than only assessing the value of single medications as a part of the treatment plan.

In addition to reviewing past and current treatments, including other nonpharmacological treatments (e.g., ECT, TMS, light therapy), it is important to determine whether the patient has co-occurring psychiatric symptoms or disorders that warrant medication treatment (see the subsection

"Addressing Co-occurring Psychiatric Disorders" in Statement 3). Although patients with BPD often have co-occurring psychiatric disorders, such as mood disorders, PTSD, anxiety disorders, eating disorders, ADHD, SUDs, and other personality disorders (Choi-Kain et al. 2022; Friborg et al. 2014; Geluk Rouwhorst et al. 2023; Grant et al. 2016; Gunderson et al. 2014; Keuroghlian et al. 2015; Leichsenring et al. 2011; Lenzenweger et al. 2007; McDermid et al. 2015; McGlashan et al. 2000; Miller et al. 2022; Momen et al. 2022; Santo et al. 2022; Tate et al. 2022; Trull et al. 2018; Zanarini et al. 2004a, 2010, 2019; Zimmerman et al. 2017), they also may exhibit symptoms such as impulsivity or mood dysregulation that are a reflection of BPD and not indicative of a co-occurring disorder. A careful history, including a family history of psychiatric illness and a longitudinal history of psychiatric symptoms or episodes, will facilitate appropriate diagnosis of co-occurring conditions when they are present without overdiagnosing (and overtreating) co-occurring conditions when they are not present.

Statement 7 – Pharmacotherapy Principles

APA *suggests* (2C) that any psychotropic medication treatment of borderline personality disorder be time-limited, aimed at addressing a specific measurable target symptom, and adjunctive to psychotherapy.

Implementation

Despite the lack of evidence in support of medication treatment from clinical trials (see Appendix C, Statement 7, and Appendix D; Gartlehner et al. 2021; Stoffers-Winterling et al. 2022), there may be circumstances in which treatment with a medication may be considered on clinical grounds. For example, medication to address co-occurring disorders will generally be appropriate to use (see the subsection "Addressing Co-occurring Psychiatric Disorders" in Statement 3). In other circumstances, pharmacotherapy may be used on a time-limited basis as an adjunct to psychotherapy for BPD and may help diminish symptoms such as affective instability, impulsivity, or psychotic-like symptoms in individual patients, helping them to remain engaged in treatment or reducing short-term risks of self-harm.

Selection of a medication, if one appears to be appropriate, will depend on the BPD symptom or symptoms being targeted or on the typical recommended treatments for a co-occurring condition. For example, in a patient with co-occurring MDD or OCD, SSRIs may be appropriate to use. A low dosage of a second-generation antipsychotic medication may be used for treatment of BPD symptoms in patients with psychosis, high levels of impulsivity, or agitation (Bohus et al. 2021). For extremely ill hospitalized patients with BPD (with or without psychotic symptoms), clozapine may be considered based on case reports, naturalistic data, and a small clinical trial (Chengappa et al. 1999; Crawford et al. 2022; Rohde et al. 2018). Anticonvulsant mood-stabilizing medications are sometimes used but have limited evidence of efficacy in individuals with BPD without co-occurring mood disorders (Gartlehner et al. 2021; Crawford et al. 2018). Use of benzodiazepines is not generally recommended because of the potential for greater impulsivity or disinhibition as well as the potential for misuse or the development of dependence (Leichsenring et al. 2023; Lieslehto et al. 2023; Pascual et al. 2023). Decisions about medication should also consider potential risks of toxicity in overdose or potential for misuse, particularly in individuals with a co-occurring SUD. In addition, before treating a co-occurring disorder, a thorough assessment is needed to establish the diagnosis and to determine the target symptoms for ongoing monitoring.

Prior to prescribing a medication, it is important to educate patients about the adjunctive nature of the medication in treating BPD symptoms and its potential benefits and adverse effects. In particular, medications would not be expected to affect the core features of BPD. Also, the response of co-occurring conditions to medications may be less in individuals who also have BPD. Overreliance on medication can send the erroneous message that emotional responses can be addressed by pharmacotherapy. Frequent dosage escalation or medication changes in response to crises or transient mood states are also problematic and rarely effective. Potential adverse effects of specific medications should be reviewed prior to treatment initiation. Examples include risk of metabolic syndrome, weight gain, extrapyramidal side effects, or tardive dyskinesia with antipsychotic agents; risk of neural tube defects with divalproex use early in pregnancy; risk of polycystic ovary disease with divalproex in individuals with ovaries; risk of Stevens-Johnson syndrome with lamotrigine; and cognitive effects with topiramate. In adolescents, clinical trials of medications to treat BPD have not been conducted, and side effects of medications may be more problematic.

If a medication is started, the duration of treatment should be time limited, with tapering and discontinuation of the medication, if possible, once symptoms have stabilized. While treatment is occurring, however, patients should receive any monitoring that is necessary for the specific medication (e.g., serum levels for some anticonvulsants, metabolic monitoring for antipsychotics).

Communication with other members of the treatment team is an essential aspect of decision-making about medications. Treatment team members and other collateral sources of information (e.g., family members) can provide ongoing observations about symptom response, in addition to direct observation and feedback from the patient. It is also important to communicate with other health professionals, such as primary care clinicians, who may be unaware of the complexities of prescribing medications to individuals with BPD and may inadvertently prescribe unwarranted medications.

Statement 8 – Pharmacotherapy Review

APA *recommends* **(1C)** that a patient with borderline personality disorder receive a review and reconciliation of their medications at least every 6 months to assess the effectiveness of treatment and identify medications that warrant tapering or discontinuation.

Implementation

Appropriate use of pharmacotherapy for BPD includes prescribing as few medications as possible, using medication as an adjunct to treatment with psychotherapy, and selecting medications based on their ability to target specific and prominent symptom clusters (Gartlehner et al. 2021; Yadav 2020). Continuous review and reconciliation of medications is critical for avoiding or mitigating prolonged and unnecessary exposure to pharmacotherapy as well as inappropriate polypharmacy (Bridler et al. 2015; Gartlehner et al. 2021; Paris 2015; Romanowicz et al. 2020; Shapiro-Thompson and Fineberg 2022; Soler et al. 2022; Starcevic and Janca 2018). Medication reconciliation is a recommended best practice in hospital as well as outpatient settings (Institute for Safe Medication Practice 2023; The Joint Commission 2022).

Medication review has been suggested as an important part of optimizing therapeutic benefit for patients with BPD and should involve a structured, critical assessment of all medications prescribed, including among patients also participating in psychotherapy (Kadra-Scalzo et al. 2021). It is especially useful following stabilization of an acute crisis because this is often a precipitating event that prompts medication initiation, and once resolved, might preclude the need for continued pharmacotherapy (Starcevic and Janca 2018). Medication monitoring and review is an important strategy for early identification of drug-drug interactions and adverse reactions, the latter of which could lead to symptom exacerbation (e.g., use of benzodiazepines to reduce anxiety may exacerbate disinhibition and cognitive deficits) (Fineberg et al. 2019). Medication review is also necessary given the natural course of BPD, wherein symptoms fluctuate in intensity and frequency and may remit rapidly (Fineberg et al. 2019; Videler et al. 2019). In addition, patients may improve with psychotherapy and no longer require the same medications or medication dosages. Thus, patients taking medication need to be monitored carefully and routinely to determine treatment response and taper or discontinue as needed (Fineberg et al. 2019). Ongoing reevaluation of the risks and benefits of a patient's current medication should continue throughout treatment, especially given that some symptoms may resolve spontaneously (Ripoll 2013).

Appropriate use of pharmacotherapy for patients with BPD should also include a plan for deprescribing, such as tapering strategies and ongoing monitoring for changes in clinical presentation and adverse reactions (Fineberg et al. 2019; Shapiro-Thompson and Fineberg 2022). An effective plan for deprescribing includes making a list of medications—such as dosage, route of administration, duration, expected benefits, adverse reactions, and potential for withdrawal symptoms with discontinuation—and working collaboratively with the patient to weigh the risks and benefits of tapering or discontinuing the medication (Chanen and Thompson 2016; Fineberg et al. 2019).

Areas for Further Research

Methodological Issues

Our ability to draw clinically meaningful conclusions and conduct meta-analyses from research on BPD would be augmented by improvements in the design of studies. Specific steps that could be taken might include

- Improving the generalizability of study populations in terms of factors such as age, sex/gender, sexual orientation, race, ethnicity, culture, social determinants, presence of co-occurring conditions, illness severity, and risk of suicidal, aggressive, or self-harming behaviors.
- Enhancing study recruitment approaches and using a priori specification of analyses to obtain data on treatment effects in subgroups that have been underrepresented in prior research (e.g., inpatients; older individuals; individuals with multiple psychiatric or physical health conditions; individuals with severe and/or persistent illness; diverse samples of individuals in terms of sex/gender, sexual orientation, race, ethnicity, culture, neurodiversity, and social determinants).
- Developing approaches to data collection and transparent reporting of sociodemographic factors to facilitate pooling of data from multiple studies and to permit assessment of treatment effects in subgroups that have been underrepresented in previous research.
- Standardizing definitions for and collection of key data elements and outcome variables, insofar as possible.
- Incorporating individuals with lived experience into identification of data elements and outcome variables to ensure that research is assessing factors of importance to patients.
- Standardizing information, insofar as possible, on patient characteristics that are important to risk adjustment of outcomes (e.g., age at illness onset, illness duration and severity, presence of specific symptoms or symptom clusters, type and frequency of self-harming behaviors, co-occurring conditions).
- Collecting data on possible common mechanisms of psychotherapies (e.g., therapeutic alliance, therapist characteristics) in addition to elements that are hypothesized to relate to mechanisms of a specific psychotherapeutic approach.
- Reporting diagnostic information using both DSM-5-TR categorical diagnoses and the AMPD.
- Integrating dimensional measures of AMPD and symptom domains of BPD (e.g., impulsivity, affect dysregulation) into clinical trial design.
- Providing detailed information on processes used for random assignment and masking or blinding to treatment condition.
- Reporting data separately, insofar as possible, for each diagnostic group in studies that use transdiagnostic samples.
- Augmenting self-report observations with clinician interpretation of the self-report and with direct measurements of outcome, insofar as possible.
- Ensuring that sample sizes in clinical studies are estimated a priori and are adequate to achieve statistical power.
- Ensuring that studies report data in a consistent fashion, with pre-specification of outcomes of interest.
- When observations are missing, using appropriate data analytic approaches and performing sensitivity analyses, when indicated, to determine the effects of missing data.

- Identifying instruments for measuring BPD symptoms and features that are efficient, accurate, culturally sensitive, and validated in multiple languages for measuring key categorical and dimensional outcomes; fostering standardized and consistent use of such instruments across studies.
- Identifying standardized approaches for collecting information about factors that ultimately may be useful in individualizing treatment selection (e.g., biomarkers, family history, symptom history, treatment history, personality traits, self-harming behaviors).
- Ensuring that studies identify the magnitude of change in scale scores that would constitute a clinically meaningful difference.
- Increasing collection of data on patient-centered outcomes (e.g., quality of life, social functioning, physical health, recovery) and selecting these outcomes using input from individuals with lived experience.
- Developing consensus definitions of response and remission of BPD that can be applied consistently across studies.
- Developing approaches to understanding the diversity of elements and indicators of recovery using insights from individuals with lived experience.
- Providing detailed descriptions of the characteristics of active treatments, including treatment as usual, when they are used in a comparative effectiveness study.
- For studies of new treatments or adaptations of existing treatments, using standardized versions of active comparison treatments to permit consistency in comparing treatments for non-inferiority.
- For studies of new treatments or adaptations of existing treatments, conducting comparative effectiveness studies with more than a single existing treatment to allow broader conclusions to be drawn about the relative effectiveness of different interventions.
- Ensuring that studies of new treatments, technologies, delivery system modifications, or clinical decision support systems include specific attention to health equity in implementation methods.
- Developing mechanisms such as registries for systematic collection of information on program outcomes as a complement to collecting clinical trial data.
- Incorporating approaches to study recruitment and treatment implementation to reduce the impact of placebo effects on study outcomes.
- Improving systematic collection of information on harms, including in studies of psychotherapies.
- Ensuring that studies assess longer-term treatment (e.g., at least 1 year) as well as long-term follow-up assessments (e.g., 3–5 years) to identify possible long-term harms and patterns of relapse after treatment completion.

Research Topics

Prevention, Screening, and Assessment

- Identify risk factors for development of BPD that could be used in defining subgroups of adolescents or adults who warrant prospective screening or could benefit from preventive interventions.
- Determine whether patient characteristics and symptoms can be used to identify adolescents or adults who would benefit from early intervention to prevent onset of BPD.
- Determine whether specific approaches to prevention (e.g., in high-risk adolescents) are associated with benefits on patient-oriented outcomes.
- Determine whether identification of BPD using targeted screening is associated with benefits on patient-oriented outcomes in adolescents and adults.

- Determine circumstances in which the AMPD is more useful than a categorical diagnosis of BPD or in which a categorical diagnosis of BPD is more useful than the AMPD.
- Determine whether additional screening, assessment, or longitudinal rating scales need to be developed for BPD to ensure that their scores have reliability and can be interpreted as measures of a specific construct or outcome among a broad range of ages, genders, cultures, languages, symptom patterns, settings, treatment approaches, and diagnostic models (e.g., categorical, alternative model).

Treatment Planning

- Determine ways to optimize short- and long-term patient outcomes in adolescents and adults, including recovery, using factors and approaches such as
  - Early identification and intervention
  - "Stepped-care" or clinical staging approaches that start with less intensive treatment and shift to more intensive interventions, as needed, to achieve recovery
  - Telehealth (individual, group, and family)
  - Setting specific interventions (e.g., emergency, inpatient, long-term care)
  - Large-scale data analytics and predictive algorithms
  - Self-help and guided self-help approaches, including groups, manual-based approaches, or computer-based programs (including Web-based, phone applications, chatbots, and other modalities)
  - Family/caregiver interventions, including support groups and psychoeducation
  - Involving certified peer support specialists as part of the multidisciplinary team
  - Modifying treatment to improve physical health and address co-occurring health conditions, including substance-related and addictive disorders and other psychiatric disorders
  - Modifying treatment to address significant symptoms such as suicidal ideas and behaviors, NSSI, aggressive behavior, anger, mood lability, or anxiety
  - Modifying treatment to address attachment-related issues or traumatic experiences, including adverse childhood experiences
  - Modifying treatment to address development-related issues in adolescents and emerging adults
  - Developing new treatments to target key aspects of personality in BPD.
- Identify clinical indicators, biomarkers, and other factors that can help in individualizing treatment selection, frequency, and duration to achieve optimal patient outcomes in adolescents and adults.
- Identify clinical indicators, biomarkers, and other factors that can help in determining an optimal sequence of treatments, if an initial therapeutic modality is not associated with response or recovery.
- Identify approaches to individualizing treatment selection and delivery to optimize outcomes for individuals of different ages, developmental stages, sexes, genders, races, ethnicities, and cultural groups, among other individual facets.
- Obtain additional evidence in adolescents and adults on the optimal duration and frequency of treatments in relation to the severity of patient symptoms and other clinical variables.
- Obtain additional evidence in adolescents and adults on novel or existing psychotherapies (e.g., interpersonal psychotherapy, acceptance and commitment therapy, DDP) in the treatment of BPD.
- Obtain additional evidence in adolescents and adults on novel or existing psychotherapies in patients with common co-occurring disorders (e.g., PTSD, SUD, depression).
- Obtain evidence on emerging therapeutic approaches such as psychedelic- or MDMA-assisted psychotherapy, which may facilitate the psychotherapeutic process by generating greater openness and self-compassion.

- Obtain additional evidence in adolescents and adults on novel or existing pharmacotherapies in the treatment of BPD.
- Obtain additional evidence in adolescents and adults on novel or existing neurostimulation therapies, such as TMS, in the treatment of BPD.
- Conduct additional studies on the comparative effectiveness of psychotherapies and other interventions to treat BPD in adolescents and adults.
- Identify and standardize several effective psychotherapies for BPD in adults and adolescents that can then be used in a consistent fashion as an active comparator in comparative effectiveness studies.
- Conduct additional RCTs of treatment in adolescents and emerging adults.
- Identify optimal approaches to providing multidisciplinary team–based care of BPD in adolescents and adults with quantification of staff training and supervision requirements, cost-effectiveness, and program sustainability.
- Determine the circumstances in which "bundled" treatment programs are appropriate to use in adolescents and adults with BPD, including the elements of these programs that enhance patient outcomes.
- Identify clinical considerations in assessment and monitoring as well as optimal approaches to providing treatment to individuals with BPD who wish to become pregnant, are pregnant, or are breastfeeding.
- Determine which factors can be used in selecting an optimal treatment setting for adolescents and adults with BPD.
- Determine optimal monitoring frequencies and approaches to detect treatment-related benefits and adverse effects for adolescents and adults with BPD.
- Develop approaches to care that reduce relapse and avoid discontinuities in care for adolescents and adults with BPD.
- Identify the treatment elements and approaches that are viewed as most and least helpful by adolescents and adults who have responded to treatment of BPD.
- Identify differences in the characteristics of patients who seek or receive treatment with psychotherapy, pharmacotherapy, or both.
- Identify methods that will allow information from mobile technologies, wearable technology, and large-scale data analytics to inform assessment, treatment, and future research.
- Identify approaches to redesigning workflows and models of care delivery to improve the use of best practices and reduce inequities in the care of adolescents and adults with BPD.
- Determine the ways in which health system factors and treatment delivery characteristics influence patient outcomes for adolescents and adults with BPD.
- Develop approaches to the dissemination of training in effective psychotherapies.

Ethical Issues in BPD Assessment and Treatment

- Determine approaches for including individuals with lived experience in informing research goals, designs, methodologies, and interpretation, among other roles.
- Determine approaches for including family members or other caregivers of individuals with BPD in informing research goals, designs, methodologies, and interpretation, among other roles.
- Determine the optimal approaches to assess capacity to accept or decline treatment in patients with BPD.
- Determine optimal approaches (e.g., verbal communications, electronic information sharing via patient portals or open notes) for involving family in treatment while also protecting the privacy and confidentiality of adolescents and emerging adults.
- Identify ways in which social media influences BPD symptoms and treatment engagement in adolescents and adults.

- Determine whether specific policy recommendations, regulatory requirements, or adjustments to social media algorithms can reduce the deleterious effects of social media in adolescents and adults who have BPD.
- Identify ways in which risk factors, prevention, assessment, treatment, and outcomes of individuals with BPD are affected by internalized stigma and by biases and discrimination of society and health care professionals related to factors such as BPD and co-occurring diagnoses, physical health symptoms or conditions, age, sex/gender, sexual orientation, race, ethnicity, culture, and social determinants.
- Identify effective approaches to reducing and eliminating health disparities due to bias and discrimination in the assessment and treatment of adolescents and adults with BPD.
- Determine whether specific policy recommendations, regulatory requirements, or health care service delivery interventions can reduce disparities in access to care based on factors such as age, sex/gender, sexual orientation, race, ethnicity, culture, and social determinants as well as insurance status and geographical location.

Guideline Development Process

This guideline was developed using a process intended to meet standards of the Institute of Medicine (2011; now known as the National Academy of Medicine). The process is fully described in a document available on the APA Web site at: www.psychiatry.org/psychiatrists/practice/clinical-practice-guidelines/guideline-development-process.

Management of Potential Conflicts of Interest

Members of the Guideline Writing Group (GWG) are required to disclose all potential conflicts of interest before appointment, before and during guideline development, and upon publication. If any potential conflicts are found or disclosed during the guideline development process, the member must recuse themself from any related discussion and voting on a related recommendation. The members of both the GWG and the Systematic Review Group (SRG) reported no conflicts of interest. The Disclosures section includes more detailed disclosure information for each GWG and SRG member involved in the guideline's development.

Guideline Writing Group Composition

The GWG was initially composed of six psychiatrists with general research and clinical expertise (G.A.K., J.M.A., S.B., J.M.L., R.M., M.S.). This non-topic-specific group was intended to provide diverse and balanced views on the guideline topic to minimize potential bias. Three psychiatrists (L.C.-K., K.J.N., J.M.O.) and one psychologist (C.S.) were added to provide subject matter expertise in BPD. One fellow (A.D.) was involved in the guideline development process. The vice-chair of the GWG (L.J.F.) provided methodological expertise on such topics as appraising the strength of research evidence. The GWG was also diverse and balanced with respect to other characteristics, such as geographical location and demographic background. Emotions Matter and National Council for Mental Wellbeing reviewed the draft and provided perspectives from patients, families, and other care partners.

Systematic Review Methodology

The methods for this systematic review follow the Agency for Healthcare Research and Quality (AHRQ) Methods Guide for Effectiveness and Comparative Effectiveness Reviews (available at www.effectivehealthcare.ahrq.gov/methodsguide.cfm) and the Preferred Reporting Items for Systematic Reviews and Meta-Analyses (PRISMA) checklist (Moher et al. 2015). The final protocol of this review was registered on PROSPERO (Registration #: CRD42020194098). All methods and analyses were determined a priori.

This guideline is based on an initial systematic search of available research evidence conducted by Dr. Evidence (Santa Monica, CA) using the DOC Data 2.0 software platform, and an updated search conducted by RTI. The systematic search of available research evidence used MEDLINE, Cochrane Library, EMBASE, and PsycINFO databases, with specific search terms and limits as described in Appendix B. Results covered the period from the start of each database to June 15, 2020, with additional searches in MEDLINE and PsycINFO through September 24, 2021. Search strategies used a variety of terms, medical subject headings (MeSH), and major headings and were limited to English-language and human-only studies (see Appendix B). Case reports, comments, editorials, and letters were excluded. To minimize retrieval bias, we manually searched reference lists of landmark studies and background articles on this topic for relevant citations that electronic searches might have missed.

Studies were included if participants were 13 years of age or older and diagnosed with BPD as defined by DSM-IV, DSM-IV-TR, DSM-5 (Section II or Section III), or ICD-10, as applicable. Interventions of interest included psychotherapies, pharmacotherapies, and other interventions. Comparator conditions included active interventions, placebo, treatment as usual, waiting-list controls, or GPM. Multiple outcomes were included related to key symptoms and domains of BPD, functioning, quality of life, adverse effects, and study withdrawal rates, among others (see Appendix B). Studies were excluded if BPD did not account for at least 75% of the total sample. Other exclusion criteria included small sample size ($N<50$ for nonrandomized clinical trials or observational studies), lack of a comparator group, short treatment duration (<8 weeks), or studies done outside of very high Human Development Index (HDI) countries. Citations to registry links, abstracts, and proceedings were not included unless also published in a peer-reviewed journal because they did not include sufficient information to evaluate the risk of bias of the study.

For each trial identified for inclusion from the search, detailed information was extracted by RTI, with processes that included verifications and quality checks on data extraction. In addition to specific information about each reported outcome, extracted information included citation; study design; treatment arms (including dosages, sample sizes); co-intervention, if applicable; trial duration and follow-up duration, if applicable; country; setting; funding source; sample characteristics (e.g., mean age, % non-White, % female, % with co-occurring condition); and rates of attrition, among other data elements. Summary tables (see Appendix D and Appendix G) include specific details for each study identified for inclusion from the literature search. Factors relevant to risk of bias were also identified for each RCT that contributed to a guideline statement. Risk of bias was determined using the Cochrane Risk of Bias 2.0 tool (Sterne et al. 2019), and ratings are included in summary tables (see Appendix D), with specific factors contributing to the risk of bias for each study shown in Appendix E (McGuinness and Higgins 2021).

Available guidelines from other organizations were also reviewed (see Appendix F) (Canadian Agency for Drugs and Technologies in Health 2018; Finnish Medical Society Duodecim 2020; Herpertz et al. 2007; National Health and Medical Research Council 2012; National Institute for Health and Care Excellence 2009; Simonsen et al. 2019).

Rating the Strength of Supporting Research Evidence

Strength of supporting research evidence describes the level of confidence that findings from scientific observation and testing of an effect of an intervention reflect the true effect. Confidence is enhanced by such factors as rigorous study design and minimal potential for study bias.

Ratings were determined, in accordance with the AHRQ's *Methods Guide for Effectiveness and Comparative Effectiveness Reviews* (Agency for Healthcare Research and Quality 2014), by the methodologist (L.J.F.) and reviewed by members of the SRG and GWG. Available clinical trials were assessed across four primary domains: risk of bias, consistency of findings across studies, directness of the effect on a specific health outcome, and precision of the estimate of effect.

The ratings are defined as follows:

- High (denoted by the letter A) = High confidence that the evidence reflects the true effect. Further research is very unlikely to change our confidence in the estimate of effect.

- Moderate (denoted by the letter B) = Moderate confidence that the evidence reflects the true effect. Further research may change our confidence in the estimate of effect and may change the estimate.
- Low (denoted by the letter C) = Low confidence that the evidence reflects the true effect. Further research is likely to change our confidence in the estimate of effect and is likely to change the estimate.

The AHRQ has an additional category of *insufficient* for evidence that is unavailable or does not permit estimation of an effect. The APA uses the *low* rating when evidence is insufficient because there is low confidence in the conclusion, and further research, if conducted, would likely change the estimated effect or confidence in the estimated effect.

Rating the Strength of Guideline Statements

Each guideline statement is separately rated to indicate strength of recommendation and strength of supporting research evidence. *Strength of recommendation* describes the level of confidence that potential benefits of an intervention outweigh potential harms. This level of confidence is informed by available evidence, which includes evidence from clinical trials as well as expert opinion and patient values and preferences. As described earlier in "Rating the Strength of Supporting Research Evidence," this rating is a consensus judgment of the authors of the guideline.

There are two possible ratings: recommendation or suggestion. A *recommendation* (denoted by the numeral 1 after the guideline statement) indicates confidence that the benefits of the intervention clearly outweigh the harms. A *suggestion* (denoted by the numeral 2 after the guideline statement) indicates greater uncertainty. Although the benefits of the statement are still viewed as outweighing the harms, the balance of benefits and harms is more difficult to judge, or either the benefits or the harms may be less clear. With a suggestion, patient values and preferences may be more variable, and this can influence the clinical decision that is ultimately made. These strengths of recommendation correspond to ratings of *strong* or *weak* (also termed *conditional*) as defined under the GRADE method for rating recommendations in clinical practice guidelines (described in publications such as Guyatt et al. 2008 and others available on the Web site of the GRADE Working Group at www.gradeworkinggroup.org).

When a negative statement is made, ratings of strength of recommendation should be understood as meaning the inverse of the above (e.g., *recommendation* indicates confidence that harms clearly outweigh benefits).

The GWG determined ratings of the strength of the guideline statement by a modified Delphi method using blind iterative voting and discussion. For the GWG members to be able to ask for clarifications about the evidence, the wording of statements, or the process, the vice-chair of the GWG served as a resource and did not vote on statements. The chair and other formally appointed GWG members were eligible to vote.

In weighing potential benefits and harms, GWG members considered the strength of supporting research evidence, their own clinical experiences and opinions, and patient preferences. For recommendations, at least 9 out of 10 members must have voted to recommend the intervention or assessment after five rounds of voting, and at most one member was allowed to vote other than "recommend" for the intervention or assessment. On the basis of the discussion among the GWG members, adjustments to the wording of recommendations could be made between the voting rounds. If this level of consensus was not achieved, the GWG could have agreed to make a suggestion rather than a recommendation. No suggestion or statement could have been made if three or more members voted "no statement." Differences of opinion within the GWG about ratings of strength of recommendation, if any, are described in the subsection "Balancing of Potential Benefits and Harms" for each statement in Appendix F.

Use of Guidelines to Enhance Quality of Care

Clinical practice guidelines can help enhance quality by synthesizing available research evidence and delineating recommendations for care on the basis of the available evidence. In some circumstances, practice guideline recommendations will be appropriate to use in developing quality measures. Guideline statements can also be used in other ways, such as for educational activities or electronic clinical decision support, to enhance the quality of care that patients receive. Furthermore, when availability of services is a major barrier to implementing guideline recommendations, improved tracking of service availability and program development initiatives may need to be implemented by health organizations, health insurance plans, federal or state agencies, or other regulatory programs.

Typically, guideline recommendations that are chosen for development into quality measures will advance one or more aims of the Institute of Medicine's report *Crossing the Quality Chasm* (Institute of Medicine 2001) and the ongoing work guided by the AHRQ-led National Quality Strategy by facilitating care that is safe, effective, patient-centered, timely, efficient, and equitable. To achieve these aims, a broad range of quality measures (Watkins et al. 2015) is needed that spans the entire continuum of care (e.g., prevention, screening, assessment, treatment, continuing care), addresses the different levels of the health system hierarchy (e.g., system-wide, organization, program/department, individual clinicians), and includes measures of different types (e.g., process, outcome, patient-centered experience). Emphasis is also needed on factors that influence the dissemination and adoption of evidence-based practices (Drake et al. 2008; Greenhalgh et al. 2004; Horvitz-Lennon et al. 2009a).

Measure development is complex and requires detailed development of specification and pilot testing (Center for Health Policy/Center for Primary Care and Outcomes Research and Battelle Memorial Institute 2011; Fernandes-Taylor and Harris 2012; Iyer et al. 2016; Pincus et al. 2016; Watkins et al. 2011). Generally, however, measure development should be guided by the available evidence and focused on measures that are broadly relevant and meaningful to patients, clinicians, and policy makers. Measure feasibility is another crucial aspect of measure development but is often decided based on current data availability, which limits opportunities for development of novel measurement concepts. Furthermore, innovation in workflow and data collection systems can benefit from looking beyond practical limitations in the early development stages in order to foster development of meaningful measures.

Often, quality measures will focus on gaps in care or on care processes and outcomes that have significant variability across specialties, health care settings, geographical areas, or patients' demographic characteristics. Administrative databases, registries, and data from electronic health records can help identify gaps in care and key domains that would benefit from performance improvements (Acevedo et al. 2015; Patel et al. 2015; Watkins et al. 2016). Nevertheless, for some guideline statements, evidence of practice gaps or variability will be based on anecdotal observations if the typical practices of psychiatrists and other health professionals are unknown. Variability in the use of guideline-recommended approaches may reflect appropriate differences that are tailored to the patient's preferences, treatment of co-occurring illnesses, or other clinical circumstances that may not have been studied in the available research. On the other hand, variability may indicate a need to strengthen clinician knowledge or to address other barriers to adoption of best practices (Drake et al. 2008; Greenhalgh et al. 2004; Horvitz-Lennon et al. 2009a). When performance is compared among organizations, variability may reflect a need for quality improvement initiatives to improve overall outcomes but could also reflect case-mix differences such as socioeconomic factors or the prevalence of co-occurring illnesses.

When a guideline recommendation is considered for development into a quality measure, it must be possible to define the applicable patient group (i.e., the denominator) and the clinical action or outcome of interest that is measured (i.e., the numerator) in validated, clear, and quantifiable terms. Furthermore, the health system's or clinician's performance on the measure must be readily ascertained from chart review, patient-reported outcome measures, registries, or administrative data. Documentation of quality measures can be challenging, and, depending on the practice setting, can pose practical barriers to meaningful interpretation of quality measures based on guideline recommendations. For example, when recommendations relate to patient assessment or treatment selection, clinical judgment may need to be used to determine whether the clinician has addressed the factors that merit emphasis for an individual patient. In other circumstances, standardized instruments can facilitate quality measurement reporting, but it is difficult to assess the appropriateness of clinical judgment in a validated, standardized manner. Furthermore, utilization of standardized assessments remains low (Fortney et al. 2017), and clinical findings are not routinely documented in a standardized format. Many clinicians appropriately use free text prose to describe symptoms, response to treatment, discussions with family, plans of treatment, and other aspects of care and clinical decision-making. Reviewing these free text records for measurement purposes would be impractical, and it would be difficult to hold clinicians accountable to such measures without significant increases in electronic medical record use and advances in natural language processing technology.

Conceptually, quality measures can be developed for purposes of accountability, for internal or health system–based quality improvement, or both. Accountability measures require clinicians to report their rate of performance of a specified process, intermediate outcome, or outcome in a specified group of patients. Because these data are used to determine financial incentives or penalties based on performance, accountability measures must be scientifically validated, have a strong evidence base, and fill gaps in care. In contrast, internal or health system–based quality improvement measures are typically designed by and for individual providers, health systems, or payers. They typically focus on measurements that can suggest ways for clinicians or administrators to improve efficiency and delivery of services within a particular setting. Internal or health system–based quality improvement programs may or may not link performance with payment, and, in general, these measures are not subject to strict testing and validation requirements. Quality improvement activities, including performance measures derived from these guidelines, should yield improvements in quality of care to justify any clinician burden (e.g., documentation burden) or related administrative costs (e.g., for manual extraction of data from charts, for modifications of electronic medical record systems to capture required data elements). Possible unintended consequences of any derived measures would also need to be addressed in testing of a fully specified measure in a variety of practice settings. For example, highly specified measures may lead to overuse of standardized language that does not accurately reflect what has occurred in practice. If multiple discrete fields are used to capture information on a paper or electronic record form, data will be easily retrievable and reportable, but oversimplification is a possible unintended consequence of measurement. Just as guideline developers must balance the benefits and harms of a particular guideline recommendation, developers of performance measures must weigh the potential benefits, burdens, and unintended consequences of optimizing quality measure design and testing.

External Review

This guideline was made available for review June–July 2023 by the APA membership, scientific and clinical experts, allied organizations, and the public. In addition, a number of patient advocacy organizations were invited for input. Forty-seven individuals and 17 organizations submitted comments on the guideline (see the chapter "Individuals and Organizations That Submitted Comments" for a list of the names). The chair and vice-chair of the GWG reviewed and addressed all comments received; substantive issues were reviewed by the GWG.

Funding and Approval

This guideline development project was funded and supported by the APA without any involvement of industry or external funding. The guideline was submitted to the APA Assembly and APA Board of Trustees and approved on November 4, 2023, and December 9, 2023, respectively.

References

Acevedo A, Garnick DW, Dunigan R, et al: Performance measures and racial/ethnic disparities in the treatment of substance use disorders. J Stud Alcohol Drugs 76(1):57–67, 2015 25486394

ACOG Committee on Practice Bulletins—Obstetrics: ACOG Practice Bulletin: Clinical management guidelines for obstetrician-gynecologists number 92, April 2008: use of psychiatric medications during pregnancy and lactation. Obstet Gynecol 111(4):1001–1020, 2008 18378767

Agency for Healthcare Research and Quality: Methods Guide for Effectiveness and Comparative Effectiveness Reviews (AHRQ Publ No 10[14]-EHC063-EF). Rockville, MD, Agency for Healthcare Research and Quality, 2014

Aggarwal NK, Lewis-Fernández R: An introduction to the Cultural Formulation Interview. Focus 13(4):426–431, 2015 32015732

Allen JG, Frueh BC, Ellis TE, et al: Integrating outcomes assessment and research into clinical care in inpatient adult psychiatric treatment. Bull Menninger Clin 73(4):259–295, 2009 20025425

Al-Rousan T, Rubenstein L, Sieleni B, et al: Inside the nation's largest mental health institution: a prevalence study in a state prison system. BMC Public Health 17(1):342, 2017 28427371

Al-Shamali HF, Winkler O, Talarico F, et al: A systematic scoping review of dissociation in borderline personality disorder and implications for research and clinical practice: exploring the fog. Aust N Z J Psychiatry 56(10):1252–1264, 2022 35152771

American Academy of Pediatrics, American College of Obstetricians and Gynecologists: Guidelines for Perinatal Care, 8th Edition. Elk Grove Village, IL, American Academy of Pediatrics, 2017

American College of Correctional Physicians: Restricted Housing of Mentally Ill Inmates. Marion, MA, American College of Correctional Physicians, 2013. Available at: https://accpmed.org/restricted_housing_of_mentally.php. Accessed September 22, 2019.

American College of Obstetricians and Gynecologists' Committee on Obstetric Practice, Breastfeeding Expert Work Group: Committee Opinion No. 658: Optimizing support for breastfeeding as part of obstetric practice. Obstet Gynecol 127(2):e86–e92, 2016

American College of Obstetricians and Gynecologists: ACOG Committee Opinion No. 736: Optimizing postpartum care. Obstet Gynecol 131(5):e140–e150, 2018 29683911

American Educational Research Association, American Psychological Association, National Council for Measurement in Education (ed): Standards for Educational and Psychological Testing. Washington DC, American Educational Research Association, 2014

American Medical Association Code of Medical Ethics: Opinion 1.1.5.: Terminating a Patient-Physician Relationship. Chicago, IL, American Medical Association, 2023a. Available at: https://code-medical-ethics.ama-assn.org/ethics-opinions/terminating-patient-physician-relationship. Accessed February 1, 2023.

American Medical Association Code of Medical Ethics: Opinion 2.1.3.: Withholding Information From Patients. Chicago, IL, American Medical Association, 2023b. Available at: https://code-medical-ethics.ama-assn.org/ethics-opinions/withholding-information-patients. Accessed February 1, 2023.

American Psychiatric Association: Diagnostic and Statistical Manual of Mental Disorders, 4th Edition. Washington, DC, American Psychiatric Association, 1994

American Psychiatric Association: Diagnostic and Statistical Manual of Mental Disorders, 4th Edition, Text Revision. Washington, DC, American Psychiatric Association, 2000

American Psychiatric Association: Practice guideline for the treatment of patients with borderline personality disorder. Am J Psychiatry 158(10 Suppl):1–52, 2001 11665545

American Psychiatric Association: Position Statement on Treatment of Substance Use Disorders in the Criminal Justice System. Arlington, VA, American Psychiatric Association, 2007. Available at: https://www.psychiatry.org/File%20Library/About-APA/Organization-Documents-Policies/Policies/Position-2007-Substance-Abuse-Criminal-Justice.pdf. Accessed September 22, 2019.

American Psychiatric Association: Outpatient Services for the Mentally Ill Involved in the Criminal Justice System. Arlington, VA, American Psychiatric Association, 2009. Available at: https://www.psychiatry.org/File%20 Library/Psychiatrists/Directories/Library-and-Archive/task-force-reports/tfr2009_outpatient.pdf. Accessed September 27, 2019.

American Psychiatric Association: Practice Guideline for the Treatment of Patients With Major Depressive Disorder, Third Edition. Am J Psychiatry 167(10 Suppl):1–118, 2010

American Psychiatric Association: Diagnostic and Statistical Manual of Mental Disorders, 5th Edition. Arlington, VA, American Psychiatric Association, 2013a

American Psychiatric Association: The Principles of Medical Ethics With Annotations Especially Applicable to Psychiatry, 2013 Edition. Arlington, VA, American Psychiatric Association, 2013b. Available at: https://www.psychiatry.org/File%20Library/Psychiatrists/Practice/Ethics/principles-medical-ethics.pdf. Accessed April 28, 2023.

American Psychiatric Association: WHODAS 2.0 (World Health Organization Disability Assessment Schedule 2.0): 36-item version, self-administered, in Diagnostic and Statistical Manual of Mental Disorders, 5th Edition. Arlington, VA, American Psychiatric Association, 2013c, pp 747–748

American Psychiatric Association: Practice Guidelines for the Psychiatric Evaluation of Adults, 3rd Edition. Arlington, VA, American Psychiatric Association, 2016a

American Psychiatric Association: Psychiatric Services in Correctional Facilities, 3rd Edition. Arlington, VA, American Psychiatric Association, 2016b

American Psychiatric Association: Position Statement on Segregation of Prisoners With Mental Illness. Arlington, VA, American Psychiatric Association, 2017. Available at: https://www.psychiatry.org/File%20Library/About-APA/Organization-Documents-Policies/Policies/Position-2012-Prisoners-Segregation.pdf. Accessed September 22, 2019.

American Psychiatric Association: Position Statement on Solitary Confinement (Restricted Housing) of Juveniles. Washington, DC, American Psychiatric Association, 2018. Available at: https://www.psychiatry.org/File%20Library/About-APA/Organization-Documents-Policies/Policies/Position-2018-Solitary- Confinement-Restricted-Housing-of-Juveniles.pdf. Accessed October 3, 2019.

American Psychiatric Association: Diagnostic and Statistical Manual of Mental Disorders, 5th Edition, Text Revision. Washington, DC, American Psychiatric Association, 2022a

American Psychiatric Association: DSM-5-TR Online Assessment Measures. Washington, DC, American Psychiatric Association, 2022b. Available at: https://www.psychiatry.org/psychiatrists/practice/dsm/educational-resources/assessment-measures#section_16. Accessed August 28, 2023.

American Psychiatric Association: The American Psychiatric Association Practice Guideline for the Treatment of Patients With Eating Disorders, 4th Edition. Washington, DC, American Psychiatric Association, 2023

American Public Health Association: Solitary Confinement as a Public Health Issue. Washington, DC, American Public Health Association, 2013. Available at: https://www.apha.org/policies-and-advocacy/public-health-policy-statements/policy-database/2014/07/14/13/30/solitary-confinement-as-a-public-health-issue. Accessed September 22, 2019.

Amianto F, Ferrero A, Pierò A, et al: Supervised team management, with or without structured psychotherapy, in heavy users of a mental health service with borderline personality disorder: a two-year follow-up preliminary randomized study. BMC Psychiatry 11:181, 2011 22103890

Anderson LJ, Nuckols TK, Coles C, et al: A systematic overview of systematic reviews evaluating medication adherence interventions. Am J Health Syst Pharm 77(2):138–147, 2020 31901098

Andión Ó, Ferrer M, Matali J, et al: Effectiveness of combined individual and group dialectical behavior therapy compared to only individual dialectical behavior therapy: a preliminary study. Psychotherapy (Chic) 49(2):241–250, 2012 22642527

Andreoli A, Burnand Y, Cochennec MF, et al: Disappointed love and suicide: a randomized controlled trial of "abandonment psychotherapy" among borderline patients. J Pers Disord 30(2):271–287, 2016 26111250

Andrews JC, Schünemann HJ, Oxman AD, et al: GRADE guidelines: 15. Going from evidence to recommendation-determinants of a recommendation's direction and strength. J Clin Epidemiol 66(7):726–735, 2013 23570745

Ansell EB, Pinto A, Edelen MO, et al: The association of personality disorders with the prospective 7-year course of anxiety disorders. Psychol Med 41(5):1019–1028, 2011 20836909

Arntz A, van Genderen H: Schema Therapy for Borderline Personality Disorder, 2nd Edition. Hoboken, NJ, Wiley-Blackwell, 2021

Bach B, Tracy M: Clinical utility of the alternative model of personality disorders: a 10th year anniversary review. Personal Disord 13(4):369–379, 2022 35787123

Bachelor A: Clients' and therapists' views of the therapeutic alliance: similarities, differences and relationship to therapy outcome. Clin Psychol Psychother 20(2):118–135, 2013 22081490

Bahji A, Bach P, Danilewitz M, et al: Pharmacotherapies for adults with alcohol use disorders: a systematic review and network meta-analysis. J Addict Med 16(6):630–638, 2022 35653782

Baier AL, Kline AC, Feeny NC: Therapeutic alliance as a mediator of change: a systematic review and evaluation of research. Clin Psychol Rev 82:101921, 2020 33069096

Baillargeon J, Binswanger IA, Penn JV, et al: Psychiatric disorders and repeat incarcerations: the revolving prison door. Am J Psychiatry 166(1):103–109, 2009a 19047321

Baillargeon J, Penn JV, Thomas CR, et al: Psychiatric disorders and suicide in the nation's largest state prison system. J Am Acad Psychiatry Law 37(2):188–193, 2009b 19535556

Baillargeon J, Hoge SK, Penn JV: Addressing the challenge of community reentry among released inmates with serious mental illness. Am J Community Psychol 46(3–4):361–375, 2010 20865315

Baker J, Beazley PI: Judging personality disorder: a systematic review of clinician attitudes and responses to borderline personality disorder. J Psychiatr Pract 28(4):275–293, 2022 35797685

Bales DL, Timman R, Andrea H, et al: Effectiveness of day hospital mentalization-based treatment for patients with severe borderline personality disorder: a matched control study. Clin Psychol Psychother 22(5):409–417, 2015 25060747

Balshem H, Helfand M, Schünemann HJ, et al: GRADE guidelines: 3. Rating the quality of evidence. J Clin Epidemiol 64(4):401–406, 2011 21208779

Barker E, Kõlves K, De Leo D: Management of suicidal and self-harming behaviors in prisons: systematic literature review of evidence-based activities. Arch Suicide Res 18(3):227–240, 2014 24611725

Barnhill JW: The psychiatric interview and mental status examination, in The American Psychiatric Publishing Textbook of Psychiatry, 6th Edition. Edited by Hales RE, Yudofsky SC, Roberts LW. Washington, DC, American Psychiatric Publishing, 2014, pp 3–30

Barnicot K, Crawford M: Dialectical behaviour therapy v. mentalisation-based therapy for borderline personality disorder. Psychol Med 49(12):2060–2068, 2019 30303061

Barnicot K, Priebe S: Post-traumatic stress disorder and the outcome of dialectical behaviour therapy for borderline personality disorder. Personal Ment Health 7(3):181–190, 2013 24343961

Barnicot K, Katsakou C, Marougka S, et al: Treatment completion in psychotherapy for borderline personality disorder: a systematic review and meta-analysis. Acta Psychiatr Scand 123(5):327–338, 2011 21166785

Barnicot K, Redknap C, Coath F, et al: Patient experiences of therapy for borderline personality disorder: commonalities and differences between dialectical behaviour therapy and mentalization-based therapy and relation to outcomes. Psychol Psychother 95(1):212–233, 2022 34459086

Barr KR, Townsend ML, Grenyer BFS: Using peer workers with lived experience to support the treatment of borderline personality disorder: a qualitative study of consumer, carer and clinician perspectives. Borderline Personal Disord Emot Dysregul 7:20, 2020 32884819

Barr KR, Townsend ML, Grenyet BFS: Peer support for consumers with borderline personality disorder: a qualitative study. Adv Ment Health 20(1):74–85, 2022

Barroilhet SA, Ghaemi SN: When and how to use lithium. Acta Psychiatr Scand 142(3):161–172, 2020 32526812

Bartak A, Andrea H, Spreeuwenberg MD, et al: Effectiveness of outpatient, day hospital, and inpatient psychotherapeutic treatment for patients with Cluster B personality disorders. Psychother Psychosom 80(1):28–38, 2011 20975324

Bartels N, Crotty T: A Systems Approach to Treatment: The Borderline Personality Disorder Skill Training Manual. Winfield, IL, EID Treatment Systems, Inc, 1992

Bateman AW, Fonagy P: Mentalization-based treatment of BPD. J Pers Disord 18(1):36–51, 2004 15061343

Bateman A, Fonagy P: Randomized controlled trial of outpatient mentalization-based treatment versus structured clinical management for borderline personality disorder. Am J Psychiatry 166(12):1355–1364, 2009 19833787

Bateman A, Constantinou MP, Fonagy P, et al: Eight-year prospective follow-up of mentalization-based treatment versus structured clinical management for people with borderline personality disorder. Personal Disord 12(4):291–299, 2021 32584091

Beatson JA, Broadbear JH, Duncan C, et al: Avoiding misdiagnosis when auditory verbal hallucinations are present in borderline personality disorder. J Nerv Ment Dis 207(12):1048–1055, 2019 31790048

Bebbington P, Jakobowitz S, McKenzie N, et al: Assessing needs for psychiatric treatment in prisoners: 1. Prevalence of disorder. Soc Psychiatry Psychiatr Epidemiol 52(2):221–229, 2017 27878322

Beck E, Bo S, Jørgensen MS, et al: Mentalization-based treatment in groups for adolescents with borderline personality disorder: a randomized controlled trial. J Child Psychol Psychiatry 61(5):594–604, 2020 31702058

Bellino S, Zizza M, Rinaldi C, Bogetto F: Combined treatment of major depression in patients with borderline personality disorder: a comparison with pharmacotherapy. Can J Psychiatry 51(7):453–460, 2006 16838827

Bellino S, Zizza M, Rinaldi C, Bogetto F: Combined therapy of major depression with concomitant borderline personality disorder: comparison of interpersonal and cognitive psychotherapy. Can J Psychiatry 52(11):718–725, 2007 18399039

Bellino S, Rinaldi C, Bogetto F: Adaptation of interpersonal psychotherapy to borderline personality disorder: a comparison of combined therapy and single pharmacotherapy. Can J Psychiatry 55(2):74–81, 2010 20181302

Bender DS: The therapeutic alliance in the treatment of personality disorders. J Psychiatr Pract 11(2):73–87, 2005 15803042

Berg SH, Rørtveit K, Aase K: Suicidal patients' experiences regarding their safety during psychiatric in-patient care: a systematic review of qualitative studies. BMC Health Serv Res 17(1):73, 2017 28114936

Berg SH, Rørtveit K, Walby FA, Aase K: Safe clinical practice for patients hospitalised in mental health wards during a suicidal crisis: qualitative study of patient experiences. BMJ Open 10(11):e040088, 2020 33158829

Bernanke J, McCommon B: Training in good psychiatric management for borderline personality disorder in residency: an aide to learning supportive psychotherapy for challenging-to-treat patients. Psychodyn Psychiatry 46(2):181–200, 2018 29809114

Bhola P, Mehrotra K: Associations between countertransference reactions towards patients with borderline personality disorder and therapist experience levels and mentalization ability. Trends Psychiatry Psychother 43(2):116–125, 2021 34043903

Bianchini V, Cofini V, Curto M, et al: Dialectical behaviour therapy (DBT) for forensic psychiatric patients: an Italian pilot study. Crim Behav Ment Health 29(2):122–130, 2019 30648303

Bjureberg J, Ljótsson B, Tull MT, et al: Development and validation of a brief version of the Difficulties in Emotion Regulation Scale: the DERS-16. J Psychopathol Behav Assess 38(2):284–296, 2016 27239096

Black T: The Assessment of Suicide and Risk Inventory. Tyler Black, 2013. Available at: http://www.asari.ca. Accessed January 31, 2023.

Black DW, Blum N, Pfohl B, Hale N: Suicidal behavior in borderline personality disorder: prevalence, risk factors, prediction, and prevention. J Pers Disord 18(3):226–239, 2004 15237043

Black DW, Gunter T, Allen J, et al: Borderline personality disorder in male and female offenders newly committed to prison. Compr Psychiatry 48(5):400–405, 2007 17707246

Black DW, Blum N, McCormick B, Allen J: Systems Training for Emotional Predictability and Problem Solving (STEPPS) group treatment for offenders with borderline personality disorder. J Nerv Ment Dis 201(2):124–129, 2013 23364121

Black DW, Zanarini MC, Romine A, et al: Comparison of low and moderate dosages of extended-release quetiapine in borderline personality disorder: a randomized, double-blind, placebo-controlled trial. Am J Psychiatry 171(11):1174–1182, 2014 24968985

Black DW, Blum N, Allen J: Does response to the STEPPS program differ by sex, age, or race in offenders with borderline personality disorder? Compr Psychiatry 87:134–137, 2018 30393119

Blum N, St John D, Pfohl B, et al: Systems Training for Emotional Predictability and Problem Solving (STEPPS) for outpatients with borderline personality disorder: a randomized controlled trial and 1-year follow-up. Am J Psychiatry 165(4):468–478, 2008 18281407

Bo S, Vilmar JW, Jensen SL, et al: What works for adolescents with borderline personality disorder: towards a developmentally informed understanding and structured treatment model. Curr Opin Psychol 37:7–12, 2021 32652486

Bogenschutz MP, Nurnberg HG: Olanzapine versus placebo in the treatment of borderline personality disorder. J Clin Psychiatry 65(1):104–109, 2004 14744178

Bohus M, Haaf B, Simms T, et al: Effectiveness of inpatient dialectical behavioral therapy for borderline personality disorder: a controlled trial. Behav Res Ther 42(5):487–499, 2004 15033496

Bohus M, Limberger MF, Frank U, et al: Psychometric properties of the Borderline Symptom List (BSL). Psychopathology 40(2):126–132, 2007 17215599

Bohus M, Kleindienst N, Limberger MF, et al: The short version of the Borderline Symptom List (BSL-23): development and initial data on psychometric properties. Psychopathology 42(1):32–39, 2009 19023232

Bohus M, Dyer AS, Priebe K, et al: Dialectical behaviour therapy for post-traumatic stress disorder after childhood sexual abuse in patients with and without borderline personality disorder: a randomised controlled trial. Psychother Psychosom 82(4):221–233, 2013 23712109

Bohus M, Kleindienst N, Hahn C, et al: Dialectical behavior therapy for posttraumatic stress disorder (DBT-PTSD) compared with cognitive processing therapy (CPT) in complex presentations of PTSD in women survivors of childhood abuse: a randomized clinical trial. JAMA Psychiatry 77(12):1235–1245, 2020 32697288

Bohus M, Stoffers-Winterling J, Sharp C, et al: Borderline personality disorder. Lancet 398(10310):1528–1540, 2021 34688371

Boritz T, Barnhart R, McMain SF: The influence of posttraumatic stress disorder on treatment outcomes of patients with borderline personality disorder. J Pers Disord 30(3):395–407, 2016 26305394

Bos EH, van Wel EB, Appelo MT, et al: A randomized controlled trial of a Dutch version of systems training for emotional predictability and problem solving for borderline personality disorder. J Nerv Ment Dis 198(4):299–304, 2010 20386260

Botter L, Ten Have M, Gerritsen D, et al: Impact of borderline personality disorder traits on the association between age and health-related quality of life: a cohort study in the general population. Eur Psychiatry 64(1):e33, 2021 33896434

Bozzatello P, Bellino S: Interpersonal psychotherapy as a single treatment for borderline personality disorder: a pilot randomized-controlled study. Front Psychiatry 11:578910, 2020 33061926

Bozzatello P, Rocca P, Uscinska M, et al: Efficacy and tolerability of asenapine compared with olanzapine in borderline personality disorder: an open-label randomized controlled trial. CNS Drugs 31(9):809–819, 2017 28741044

Brand BL, Lanius RA: Chronic complex dissociative disorders and borderline personality disorder: disorders of emotion dysregulation? Borderline Personal Disord Emot Dysregul 1:13, 2014 26401297

Bridler R, Häberle A, Müller ST, et al: Psychopharmacological treatment of 2195 in-patients with borderline personality disorder: a comparison with other psychiatric disorders. Eur Neuropsychopharmacol 25(6):763–772, 2015 25907249

Brito JP, Domecq JP, Murad MH, et al: The Endocrine Society guidelines: when the confidence cart goes before the evidence horse. J Clin Endocrinol Metab 98(8):3246–3252, 2013 23783104

Burns CJ, Borah L, Terrell SM, et al: Trauma-informed care curricula for the health professions: a scoping review of best practices for design, implementation, and evaluation. Acad Med 98(3):401–409, 2023 36538661

Busch AJ, Balsis S, Morey LC, et al: Gender differences in borderline personality disorder features in an epidemiological sample of adults age 55–64: self versus informant report. J Pers Disord 30(3):419–432, 2016 26067157

Cailhol L, Roussignol B, Klein R, et al: Borderline personality disorder and rTMS: a pilot trial. Psychiatry Res 216(1):155–157, 2014 24503285

Caligor E, Kernberg OK, Clarkin JF, et al: Psychodynamic Therapy for Personality Pathology: Treating Self and Interpersonal Functioning. Washington, DC, American Psychiatric Association Publishing, 2018

Canadian Agency for Drugs and Technologies in Health: Treatment of Personality Disorders in Adults With or Without Comorbid Mental Health Conditions: Clinical Effectiveness and Guidelines. (CADTH Rapid Response Report: Summary of Abstracts). Ottawa, Canada, Canadian Agency for Drugs and Technologies in Health, February 2018. Available at: https://www.cadth.ca/sites/default/files/pdf/htis/2018/RB1199%20Personality%20Disorders%20Final.pdf. Accessed April 28, 2023.

Carlyle D, Green R, Inder M, et al: A randomized-controlled trial of mentalization-based treatment compared with structured case management for borderline personality disorder in a mainstream public health service. Front Psychiatry 11:561916, 2020 33262710

Carmona i Farrés C, Elices M, Soler J, et al: Effects of mindfulness training on borderline personality disorder: Impulsivity versus emotional dysregulation. Mindfulness 10:1243–1254, 2019a

Carmona I Farrés C, Elices M, Soler J, et al: Effects of mindfulness training on the default mode network in borderline personality disorder. Clin Psychol Psychother 26(5):562–571, 2019b 31132302

Carpenter RW, Wood PK, Trull TJ: Comorbidity of borderline personality disorder and lifetime substance use disorders in a nationally representative sample. J Pers Disord 30(3):336–350, 2016 25893556

Carter GL, Willcox CH, Lewin TJ, et al: Hunter DBT project: randomized controlled trial of dialectical behaviour therapy in women with borderline personality disorder. Aust N Z J Psychiatry 44(2):162–173, 2010 20113305

Casiano H, Katz LY, Globerman D, et al: Suicide and deliberate self-injurious behavior in juvenile correctional facilities: a review. J Can Acad Child Adolesc Psychiatry 22(2):118–124, 2013 23667357

Center for Health Policy/Center for Primary Care and Outcomes Research and Battelle Memorial Institute: Quality Indicator Measure Development, Implementation, Maintenance, and Retirement. Contract No 290-04-0020. Rockville, MD, Agency for Healthcare Research and Quality, 2011

Center for Substance Abuse Treatment: Trauma-Informed Care in Behavioral Health Services (Treatment Improvement Protocol [TIP] Series, No 57). Rockville, MD, Substance Abuse and Mental Health Services Administration, 2014

Centers for Medicare and Medicaid Services: Blueprint measure lifecycle, in Measures Management System Hub. Baltimore, MD, Centers for Medicare and Medicaid Services, March 2023. Available at: https://mmshub.cms.gov/measure-lifecycle/measure-specification/overview. Accessed May 7, 2023.

Central Institute of Mental Health: Information and Downloads: Psychosomatic Medicine and Psychotherapy. BSL-23 / BSL-95—Questionnaires. Mannheim, Germany, Central Institute of Mental Health, 2020. Available at: https://www.zi-mannheim.de/en/forschung/abteilungen-ags-institute/psm/information-and-downloads-psychosomatic-medicine-and-psychotherapy.html. Accessed January 4, 2023.

Ceresa A, Esposito CM, Buoli M: How does borderline personality disorder affect management and treatment response of patients with major depressive disorder? A comprehensive review. J Affect Disord 281:581–589, 2021 33250202

Chanen AM, Thompson KN: Prescribing and borderline personality disorder. Aust Prescr 39(2):49–53, 2016 27340322

Chanen AM, Jackson HJ, McCutcheon LK, et al: Early intervention for adolescents with borderline personality disorder using cognitive analytic therapy: randomised controlled trial. Br J Psychiatry 193(6):477–484, 2008 19043151

Chanen AM, Betts JK, Jackson H, et al: Effect of 3 forms of early intervention for young people with borderline personality disorder: the MOBY randomized clinical trial. JAMA Psychiatry 79(2):109–119, 2022 34910093

Chen EY, Brown MZ, Harned MS, et al: A comparison of borderline personality disorder with and without eating disorders. Psychiatry Res 170(1):86–90, 2009 19796824

Chen PH, Tsai SY, Chen PY, et al: Mood stabilizers and risk of all-cause, natural, and suicide mortality in bipolar disorder: a nationwide cohort study. Acta Psychiatr Scand 147(3):234–247, 2023 36367926

Cheney L, Dudas RB, Traynor JM, et al: Co-occurring autism spectrum and borderline personality disorder: an emerging clinical challenge seeking informed interventions. Harv Rev Psychiatry 31(2):83–91, 2023 36884039

Chengappa KN, Ebeling T, Kang JS, et al: Clozapine reduces severe self-mutilation and aggression in psychotic patients with borderline personality disorder. J Clin Psychiatry 60(7):477–484, 1999 10453803

Chiappini S, Picutti E, Alessi MC, et al: Efficacy of noninvasive brain stimulation on borderline personality disorder core symptoms: a systematic review. J Pers Disord 36(5):505–526, 2022 36181488

Chisolm MS, Payne JL: Management of psychotropic drugs during pregnancy. BMJ 532:h5918, 2016 26791406

Choi-Kain LW, Albert EB, Gunderson JG: Evidence-based treatments for borderline personality disorder: implementation, integration, and stepped care. Harv Rev Psychiatry 24(5):342–356, 2016 27603742

Choi-Kain LW, Finch EF, Masland SR, et al: What works in the treatment of borderline personality disorder. Curr Behav Neurosci Rep 4(1):21–30, 2017 28331780

Choi-Kain LW, Sahin Z, Traynor J: Borderline personality disorder: updates in a postpandemic world. Focus Am Psychiatr Publ 20(4):337–352, 2022 37200886

Cipriano A, Cella S, Cotrufo P: Nonsuicidal self-injury: a systematic review. Front Psychol 8:1946, 2017 29167651

Clarke DE, Wilcox HC, Miller L, et al: Feasibility and acceptability of the DSM-5 Field Trial procedures in the Johns Hopkins Community Psychiatry Programs. Int J Methods Psychiatr Res 23(2):267–278, 2014 24615761

Clarkin JF, Levy KN, Lenzenweger MF, et al: Evaluating three treatments for borderline personality disorder: a multiwave study. Am J Psychiatry 164(6):922–928, 2007 17541052

Clausen W, Watanabe-Galloway S, Bill Baerentzen M, et al: Health literacy among people with serious mental illness. Community Ment Health J 52(4):399–405, 2016 26443671

Cohen AN, Drapalski AL, Glynn SM, et al: Preferences for family involvement in care among consumers with serious mental illness. Psychiatr Serv 64(3):257–263, 2013 23242515

Cohen AN, Hamilton AB, Saks ER, et al: How occupationally high-achieving individuals with a diagnosis of schizophrenia manage their symptoms. Psychiatr Serv 68(4):324–329, 2017 27842472

Comtois KA, Carmel A: Borderline personality disorder and high utilization of inpatient psychiatric hospitalization: concordance between research and clinical diagnosis. J Behav Health Serv Res 43(2):272–280, 2016 24875431

Copeland ME: Wellness recovery action plan. Occup Ther Ment Health 17:3–4, 127–150, 2000

Cottraux J, Note ID, Boutitie F, et al: Cognitive therapy versus Rogerian supportive therapy in borderline personality disorder: two-year follow-up of a controlled pilot study. Psychother Psychosom 78(5):307–316, 2009 19628959

Council of Medical Specialty Societies: Principles for the Development of Specialty Society Clinical Guidelines. Chicago, IL, Council of Medical Specialty Societies, 2017

Courtois CA, Brown LS, Cook J, et al: Clinical Practice Guideline for the Treatment of Posttraumatic Stress Disorder (PTSD) in Adults. Washington, DC, American Psychological Association Guideline Development Panel for the Treatment of PTSD in Adults, 2017

Cowdry RW, Gardner DL: Pharmacotherapy of borderline personality disorder: alprazolam, carbamazepine, trifluoperazine, and tranylcypromine. Arch Gen Psychiatry 45(2):111–119, 1988 3276280

Crawford MJ, Sanatinia R, Barrett B, et al: The clinical effectiveness and cost-effectiveness of lamotrigine in borderline personality disorder: a randomized placebo-controlled trial. Am J Psychiatry 175(8):756–764, 2018 29621901

Crawford MJ, Leeson VC, Evans R, et al: The clinical effectiveness and cost effectiveness of clozapine for inpatients with severe borderline personality disorder (CALMED study): a randomised placebo-controlled trial. Ther Adv Psychopharmacol 12:20451253221090832, 2022 35510087

Cuijpers P, Veen SCV, Sijbrandij M, et al: Eye movement desensitization and reprocessing for mental health problems: a systematic review and meta-analysis. Cogn Behav Ther 49(3):165–180, 2020 32043428

Culina I, Fiscalini E, Martin-Soelch C, et al: The first session matters: therapist responsiveness and the therapeutic alliance in the treatment of borderline personality disorder. Clin Psychol Psychother 30(1):131–140, 2023 36066208

Davidson K, Norrie J, Tyrer P, et al: The effectiveness of cognitive behavior therapy for borderline personality disorder: results from the Borderline Personality Disorder Study of Cognitive Therapy (BOSCOT) trial. J Pers Disord 20(5):450–465, 2006 17032158

Davidson KM, Brown TM, James V, et al: Manual-assisted cognitive therapy for self-harm in personality disorder and substance misuse: a feasibility trial. Psychiatr Bull 38:108–111, 2014

de Aquino Ferreira LF, Queiroz Pereira FH, Neri Benevides AML, et al: Borderline personality disorder and sexual abuse: a systematic review. Psychiatry Res 262:70–77, 2018 29407572

de Freixo Ferreira L, Guerra C, Vieira-Coelho MA: Predictors of psychotherapy dropout in patients with borderline personality disorder: a systematic review. Clin Psychol Psychother 30(6):1324–1337, 2023 37522280

de la Fuente JM, Lotstra F: A trial of carbamazepine in borderline personality disorder. Eur Neuropsychopharmacol 4(4):479–486, 1994 7894258

De Los Reyes A, Augenstein TM, Wang M, et al: The validity of the multi-informant approach to assessing child and adolescent mental health. Psychol Bull 141(4):858–900, 2015 25915035

Dean K, Singh S, Soon YL: Decriminalizing severe mental illness by reducing risk of contact with the criminal justice system, including for forensic patients. CNS Spectr 25(5):687–700, 2020 32248861

Denning DM, Newlands RT, Gonzales A, et al: Borderline personality disorder symptoms in a community sample of sexually and gender diverse adults. J Pers Disord 36(6):701–716, 2022 36454158

Department of Veterans Affairs/Department of Defense: VA/DoD Clinical Practice Guideline for the Management of Major Depressive Disorder. Washington, DC, U.S. Government Printing Office, 2022

Department of Veterans Affairs/Department of Defense: VA/DoD Clinical Practice Guideline for Management of Posttraumatic Stress Disorder and Acute Stress Disorder. Washington, DC, U.S. Government Printing Office, 2023

DesRoches CM, Leveille S, Bell SK, et al: The views and experiences of clinicians sharing medical record notes with patients. JAMA Netw Open 3(3):e201753, 2020 32219406

Dixon LB, Holoshitz Y, Nossel I: Treatment engagement of individuals experiencing mental illness: review and update. World Psychiatry 15(1):13–20, 2016 26833597

Djulbegovic B, Trikalinos TA, Roback J, et al: Impact of quality of evidence on the strength of recommendations: an empirical study. BMC Health Serv Res 9:120, 2009 19622148

Doering S: Borderline personality disorder in patients with medical illness: a review of assessment, prevalence, and treatment options. Psychosom Med 81(7):584–594, 2019 31232916

Doering S, Hörz S, Rentrop M, et al: Transference-focused psychotherapy v. treatment by community psychotherapists for borderline personality disorder: randomised controlled trial. Br J Psychiatry 196(5):389–395, 2010 20435966

Doyle M, While D, Mok PL, et al: Suicide risk in primary care patients diagnosed with a personality disorder: a nested case control study. BMC Fam Pract 17:106, 2016 27495284

Draine J, Blank Wilson A, Metraux S, et al: The impact of mental illness status on the length of jail detention and the legal mechanism of jail release. Psychiatr Serv 61(5):458–462, 2010 20439365

Drake R, Skinner J, Goldman HH: What explains the diffusion of treatments for mental illness? Am J Psychiatry 165(11):1385–1392, 2008 18981070

Durdurak BB, Altaweel N, Upthegrove R, et al: Understanding the development of bipolar disorder and borderline personality disorder in young people: a meta-review of systematic reviews. Psychol Med 52(16):1–14, 2022 36177878

Edwards ER, Tran H, Wrobleski J, et al: Prevalence of personality disorders across veteran samples: a meta-analysis. J Pers Disord 36(3):339–358, 2022 35647770

El-Gabalawy R, Katz LY, Sareen J: Comorbidity and associated severity of borderline personality disorder and physical health conditions in a nationally representative sample. Psychosom Med 72(7):641–647, 2010 20508177

Elices M, Pascual JC, Portella MJ, et al: Impact of mindfulness training on borderline personality disorder: a randomized trial. Mindfulness 7:584–595, 2016

Ellison WD, Rosenstein LK, Morgan TA, et al: Community and clinical epidemiology of borderline personality disorder. Psychiatr Clin North Am 41(4):561–573, 2018 30447724

Emotions Matter: Emotions Matter BPD Advocacy Awareness Connection. Garden City, NY, Emotions Matter Inc, 2023a. Available at: https://emotionsmatterbpd.org. Accessed August 30, 2023.

Emotions Matter: Emotions Matter's BPD Peer Online Support Group Program. Garden City, NY, Emotions Matter Inc, 2023b. Available at: https://emotionsmatterbpd.org/peer-support-groups-information. Accessed September 2, 2023.

Epshteyn I, Mahmoud H: Enhancing mental health treatment for borderline personality disorder in corrections. J Correct Health Care 27(4):220–225, 2021 34491832

Epstein RS: Keeping Boundaries: Maintaining Safety and Integrity in the Psychotherapeutic Process. Washington, DC, American Psychiatric Publishing Inc, 1994

Farrell JM, Shaw IA, Webber MA: A schema-focused approach to group psychotherapy for outpatients with borderline personality disorder: a randomized controlled trial. J Behav Ther Exp Psychiatry 40(2):317–328, 2009 19176222

Favril L, Yu R, Hawton K, Fazel S: Risk factors for self-harm in prison: a systematic review and meta-analysis. Lancet Psychiatry 7(8):682–691, 2020 32711709

Feffer K, Lee HH, Wu W, et al: Dorsomedial prefrontal rTMS for depression in borderline personality disorder: a pilot randomized crossover trial. J Affect Disord 301:273–280, 2022 34942227

Feigenbaum JD, Fonagy P, Pilling S, et al: A real-world study of the effectiveness of DBT in the UK National Health Service. Br J Clin Psychol 51(2):121–141, 2012 22574799

Fernandes-Taylor S, Harris AH: Comparing alternative specifications of quality measures: access to pharmacotherapy for alcohol use disorders. J Subst Abuse Treat 42(1):102–107, 2012 21839604

Ferri M, Amato L, Davoli M: Alcoholics Anonymous and other 12-step programmes for alcohol dependence. Cochrane Database Syst Rev (3):CD005032, 2006 16856072

Feske U, Mulsant BH, Pilkonis PA, et al: Clinical outcome of ECT in patients with major depression and comorbid borderline personality disorder. Am J Psychiatry 161(11):2073–2080, 2004 15514409

Fineberg SK, Gupta S, Leavitt J: Collaborative deprescribing in borderline personality disorder: a narrative review. Harv Rev Psychiatry 27(2):75–86, 2019 30676404

Fineberg SK, Choi EY, Shapiro-Thompson R, et al: A pilot randomized controlled trial of ketamine in Borderline Personality Disorder. Neuropsychopharmacology 48(7):991–999, 2023 36804489

Finnish Medical Society Duodecim: Borderline personality disorder. current care summary. Duodecim Current Care Guidelines, August 6, 2020. Available at: https://www.kaypahoito.fi/en/ccs00043. Accessed April 28, 2023.

Firth J, Siddiqi N, Koyanagi A, et al: The Lancet Psychiatry Commission: a blueprint for protecting physical health in people with mental illness. Lancet Psychiatry 6(8):675–712, 2019 31324560

Fliege H, Kocalevent RD, Walter OB, et al: Three assessment tools for deliberate self-harm and suicide behavior: evaluation and psychopathological correlates. J Psychosom Res 61(1):113–121, 2006 16813853

Fonagy P, Speranza M, Luyten P, et al: ESCAP Expert Article: borderline personality disorder in adolescence: an expert research review with implications for clinical practice. Eur Child Adolesc Psychiatry 24(11):1307–1320, 2015 26271454

Ford JD, Courtois CA: Complex PTSD and borderline personality disorder. Borderline Personal Disord Emot Dysregul 8(1):16, 2021 33958001

Fornaro M, Orsolini L, Marini S, et al: The prevalence and predictors of bipolar and borderline personality disorders comorbidity: systematic review and meta-analysis. J Affect Disord 195:105–118, 2016 26881339

Fortney JC, Unützer J, Wrenn G, et al: A tipping point for measurement-based care. Psychiatr Serv 68(2):179–188, 2017 27582237

Fountoulakis KN, Tohen M, Zarate CA Jr: Lithium treatment of bipolar disorder in adults: a systematic review of randomized trials and meta-analyses. Eur Neuropsychopharmacol 54:100–115, 2022 34980362

Fowler JC, Charak R, Elhai JD, et al: Construct validity and factor structure of the Difficulties in Emotion Regulation Scale among adults with severe mental illness. J Psychiatr Res 58:175–180, 2014 25171941

Fowler JC, Clapp JD, Madan A, et al: A naturalistic longitudinal study of extended inpatient treatment for adults with borderline personality disorder: an examination of treatment response, remission and deterioration. J Affect Disord 235:323–331, 2018 29665515

Frank JD, Frank JB: Persuasion and Healing: A Comparative Study of Psychotherapy, 3rd Edition. Baltimore, MD, The Johns Hopkins University Press, 1993

Frankenburg FR, Zanarini MC: Divalproex sodium treatment of women with borderline personality disorder and bipolar II disorder: a double-blind placebo-controlled pilot study. J Clin Psychiatry 63(5):442–446, 2002 12019669

Frei-Lanter CM, Vavricka SR, Kruger TH, et al: Endoscopy for repeatedly ingested sharp foreign bodies in patients with borderline personality disorder: an international survey. Eur J Gastroenterol Hepatol 24(7):793–797, 2012 22562115

Friborg O, Martinsen EW, Martinussen M, et al: Comorbidity of personality disorders in mood disorders: a meta-analytic review of 122 studies from 1988 to 2010. J Affect Disord 152–154:1–11, 2014 24120406

Fries BE, Schmorrow A, Lang SW, et al: Symptoms and treatment of mental illness among prisoners: a study of Michigan state prisons. Int J Law Psychiatry 36(3–4):316–325, 2013 23688801

Gabbard GO, Wilkinson SM: Management of Countertransference with Borderline Patients. Lanham, MD, Jason Aronson, 2000

Gabbard GO, Kassaw KA, Perez-Garcia G: Professional boundaries in the era of the internet. Acad Psychiatry 35(3):168–174, 2011 21602438

Gaily-Luoma S, Valkonen J, Holma J, et al: How do health care services help and hinder recovery after a suicide attempt? A qualitative analysis of Finnish service user perspectives. Int J Ment Health Syst 16(1):52, 2022 36384814

García-Carmona JA, Simal-Aguado J, Campos-Navarro MP, et al: Off-label use of second-generation antipsychotics in borderline personality disorder: a comparative real-world study among oral and long-acting injectables in Spain. Int Clin Psychopharmacol 36(4):201–207, 2021 33853106

Gardner DL, Cowdry RW: Positive effects of carbamazepine on behavioral dyscontrol in borderline personality disorder. Am J Psychiatry 143(4):519–522, 1986 3513634

Gartlehner G, West SL, Mansfield AJ, et al: Clinical heterogeneity in systematic reviews and health technology assessments: synthesis of guidance documents and the literature. Int J Technol Assess Health Care 28(1):36–43, 2012 22217016

Gartlehner G, Crotty K, Kennedy S, et al: Pharmacological treatments for borderline personality disorder: a systematic review and meta-analysis. CNS Drugs 35(10):1053–1067, 2021 34495494

Geluk Rouwhorst A, Ten Have M, de Graaf R, et al: The impact of borderline personality disorder symptoms on onset and course of anxiety disorders: results of a general population study. Personal Disord 14(3):360–368, 2023 35925702

Giesen-Bloo J, van Dyck R, Spinhoven P, et al: Outpatient psychotherapy for borderline personality disorder: randomized trial of schema-focused therapy vs transference-focused psychotherapy. Arch Gen Psychiatry 63(6):649–658, 2006 16754838

Giourou E, Skokou M, Andrew SP, et al: Complex posttraumatic stress disorder: the need to consolidate a distinct clinical syndrome or to reevaluate features of psychiatric disorders following interpersonal trauma? World J Psychiatry 8(1):12–19, 2018 29568727

Glowa-Kollisch S, Kaba F, Waters A, et al: From punishment to treatment: the "Clinical Alternative to Punitive Segregation" (CAPS) program in New York City jails. Int J Environ Res Public Health 13(2):182, 2016 26848667

Goldhammer H, Crall C, Keuroghlian AS: Distinguishing and addressing gender minority stress and borderline personality symptoms. Harv Rev Psychiatry 27(5):317–325, 2019 31490187

González-González S, Marañón-González R, Hoyuela-Zatón F, et al: STEPPS for borderline personality disorder: a pragmatic trial and naturalistic comparison with noncompleters. J Pers Disord 35(6):841–856, 2021 33661018

Goodman M, Tomas IA, Temes CM, et al: Suicide attempts and self-injurious behaviours in adolescent and adult patients with borderline personality disorder. Personal Ment Health 11(3):157–163, 2017 28544496

Grambal A, Prasko J, Ociskova M, et al: Borderline personality disorder and unmet needs. Neuroendocrinol Lett 38(4):275–289, 2017 28871714

Grant BF, Chou SP, Goldstein RB, et al: Prevalence, correlates, disability, and comorbidity of DSM-IV borderline personality disorder: results from the Wave 2 National Epidemiologic Survey on Alcohol and Related Conditions. J Clin Psychiatry 69(4):533–545, 2008 18426259

Grant BF, Saha TD, Ruan WJ, et al: Epidemiology of DSM-5 drug use disorder: results from the National Epidemiologic Survey on Alcohol and Related Conditions–III. JAMA Psychiatry 73(1):39–47, 2016 26580136

Gratz KL: Measurement of deliberate self-harm: preliminary data on the Deliberate Self-Harm Inventory. J Psychopathol Behav Assess 23(4):253–263, 2001

Gratz KL, Gunderson JG: Preliminary data on an acceptance-based emotion regulation group intervention for deliberate self-harm among women with borderline personality disorder. Behav Ther 37(1):25–35, 2006 16942958

Gratz KL, Roemer L: Multidimensional assessment of emotion regulation and dysregulation: development, factor structure, and initial validation of the difficulties in emotion regulation scale. J Psychopathol Behav Assess 26(1):41–54, 2004

Gratz KL, Tull MT, Levy R: Randomized controlled trial and uncontrolled 9-month follow-up of an adjunctive emotion regulation group therapy for deliberate self-harm among women with borderline personality disorder. Psychol Med 44(10):2099–2112, 2014 23985088

Greenhalgh T, Robert G, Macfarlane F, et al: Diffusion of innovations in service organizations: systematic review and recommendations. Milbank Q 82(4):581–629, 2004 15595944

Gregory RJ: Clinical, Training, and Research Manual of Dynamic Deconstructive Psychotherapy v. 07.05.22. Syracuse, NY, Robert J. Gregory, M.D., 2022. Available at: https://www.upstate.edu/psych/pdf/manual.pdf. Accessed April 20, 2023.

Gregory RJ, Remen AL: A manual-based psychodynamic therapy for treatment-resistant borderline personality disorder. Psychotherapy (Chic) 45(1):15–27, 2008 22122362

Gregory RJ, Sachdeva S: Naturalistic outcomes of evidence-based therapies for borderline personality disorder at a medical university clinic. Am J Psychother 70(2):167–184, 2016 27329405

Gregory RJ, Chlebowski S, Kang D, et al: A controlled trial of psychodynamic psychotherapy for co-occurring borderline personality disorder and alcohol use disorder. Psychotherapy (Chic) 45(1):28–41, 2008 22122363

Gregory RJ, Remen AL, Soderberg M, et al: A controlled trial of psychodynamic psychotherapy for co-occurring borderline personality disorder and alcohol use disorder: six-month outcome. J Am Psychoanal Assoc 57(1):199–205, 2009 19270255

Gregory RJ, DeLucia-Deranja E, Mogle JA: Dynamic deconstructive psychotherapy versus optimized community care for borderline personality disorder co-occurring with alcohol use disorders: a 30-month follow-up. J Nerv Ment Dis 198(4):292–298, 2010 20386259

Gremaud-Heitz D, Riemenschneider A, Walter M, et al: Comorbid atypical depression in borderline personality disorder is common and correlated with anxiety-related psychopathology. Compr Psychiatry 55(3):650–656, 2014 24457033

Griengl H, Sendera A, Dantendorfer K: Naltrexone as a treatment of self-injurious behavior: a case report. Acta Psychiatr Scand 103(3):234–236, 2001 11240582

Grilo CM, Udo T: Association of borderline personality disorder criteria with suicide attempts among US adults. JAMA Netw Open 4(5):e219389, 2021 33974054

Gross R, Olfson M, Gameroff M, et al: Borderline personality disorder in primary care. Arch Intern Med 162(1):53–60, 2002 11784220

Guillén Botella V, García-Palacios A, Bolo Miñana S, et al: Exploring the effectiveness of dialectical behavior therapy versus systems training for emotional predictability and problem solving in a sample of patients with borderline personality disorder. J Pers Disord 35(Suppl A):21–38, 2021 32250206

Gunderson JG: Borderline personality disorder: ontogeny of a diagnosis. Am J Psychiatry 166(5):530–539, 2009 19411380

Gunderson JG, Berkowitz C: Borderline Personality Disorder Family Guidelines. Washington, NJ, National Education Alliance for Borderline Personality Disorder, 1991. Available at: https://www.borderlinepersonalitydisorder.org/family connections/family guidelines. Accessed March 1, 2023.

Gunderson JG, Stout RL, Sanislow CA, et al: New episodes and new onsets of major depression in borderline and other personality disorders. J Affect Disord 111(1):40–45, 2008 18358539

Gunderson JG, Stout RL, McGlashan TH, et al: Ten-year course of borderline personality disorder: psychopathology and function from the Collaborative Longitudinal Personality Disorders study. Arch Gen Psychiatry 68(8):827–837, 2011 21464343

Gunderson JG, Stout RL, Shea MT, et al: Interactions of borderline personality disorder and mood disorders over 10 years. J Clin Psychiatry 75(8):829–834, 2014 25007118

Gunderson J, Masland S, Choi-Kain L: Good psychiatric management: a review. Curr Opin Psychol 21:127–131, 2018 29547739

Gutheil TG: Boundary issues and personality disorders. J Psychiatr Pract 11(2):88–96, 2005 15803043

Guyatt G, Gutterman D, Baumann MH, et al: Grading strength of recommendations and quality of evidence in clinical guidelines: report from an American College of Chest Physicians Task Force. Chest 129(1):174–181, 2006 16424429

Guyatt GH, Oxman AD, Kunz R, et al: Going from evidence to recommendations. BMJ 336:1049–1051, 2008 18467413

Guyatt G, Eikelboom JW, Akl EA, et al: A guide to GRADE guidelines for the readers of JTH. J Thromb Haemost 11(8):1603–1608, 2013 23773710

Ha C, Balderas JC, Zanarini MC, et al: Psychiatric comorbidity in hospitalized adolescents with borderline personality disorder. J Clin Psychiatry 75(5):e457–e464, 2014 24922498

Hailes HP, Yu R, Danese A, et al: Long-term outcomes of childhood sexual abuse: an umbrella review. Lancet Psychiatry 6(10):830–839, 2019 31519507

Hallion LS, Steinman SA, Tolin DF, et al: Psychometric properties of the Difficulties in Emotion Regulation Scale (DERS) and its short forms in adults with emotional disorders. Front Psychol 9:539, 2018 29725312

Hamann J, Heres S: Why and how family caregivers should participate in shared decision making in mental health. Psychiatr Serv 70(5):418–421, 2019 30784381

Harding KJ, Rush AJ, Arbuckle M, et al: Measurement-based care in psychiatric practice: a policy framework for implementation. J Clin Psychiatry 72(8):1136–1143, 2011 21295000

Harford TC, Chen CM, Kerridge BT, et al: Borderline personality disorder and violence toward self and others: a national study. J Pers Disord 33(5):653–670, 2019 30307827

Harned MS, Valenstein HR: Treatment of borderline personality disorder and co-occurring anxiety disorders. F1000Prime Rep 5:15, 2013 23710329

Harned MS, Korslund KE, Linehan MM: A pilot randomized controlled trial of dialectical behavior therapy with and without the dialectical behavior therapy prolonged exposure protocol for suicidal and self-injuring women with borderline personality disorder and PTSD. Behav Res Ther 55:7–17, 2014 24562087

Harned MS, Wilks CR, Schmidt SC, et al: Improving functional outcomes in women with borderline personality disorder and PTSD by changing PTSD severity and post-traumatic cognitions. Behav Res Ther 103:53–61, 2018 29448136

Hastrup LH, Jennum P, Ibsen R, et al: Societal costs of borderline personality disorders: a matched-controlled nationwide study of patients and spouses. Acta Psychiatr Scand 140(5):458–467, 2019 31483859

Hazlehurst JM, Armstrong MJ, Sherlock M, et al: A comparative quality assessment of evidence-based clinical guidelines in endocrinology. Clin Endocrinol (Oxf) 78(2):183–190, 2013 22624723

Health Standards Organization: Leading Practices: Assessment of Suicide and Risk Inventory (ASARI) Documentation Tool. Ottawa, ON, Health Standards Organization, 2023. Available at: https://healthstandards.org/leading-practice/assessment-of-suicide-and-risk-inventory-asari-documentation-tool. Accessed February 15, 2023.

Heath LM, Laporte L, Paris J, et al: Substance misuse is associated with increased psychiatric severity among treatment-seeking individuals with borderline personality disorder. J Pers Disord 32(5):694–708, 2018a 28910215

Heath LM, Paris J, Laporte L, Gill KJ: High prevalence of physical pain among treatment-seeking individuals with borderline personality disorder. J Pers Disord 32(3):414–420, 2018b 28594632

Hein M, Mungo A, Loas G: Nonremission after electroconvulsive therapy in individuals with major depression: role of borderline personality disorder. J ECT 38(4):238–243, 2022a 35482914

Hein M, Mungo A, Loas G: Risk of relapse within 6 months associated with borderline personality disorder in major depressed individuals treated with electroconvulsive therapy. Psychiatry Res 314:114650, 2022b 35659671

Herpertz SC, Zanarini M, Schulz CS, et al: World Federation of Societies of Biological Psychiatry (WFSBP) guidelines for biological treatment of personality disorders. World J Biol Psychiatry 8(4):212–244, 2007 17963189. Available at: https://wfsbp.org/wp-content/uploads/2023/02/Guidelines_Personality_Disorders.pdf. Accessed April 28, 2023.

Herpertz SC, Matzke B, Hillmann K, et al: A mechanism-based group-psychotherapy approach to aggressive behaviour in borderline personality disorder: findings from a cluster-randomised controlled trial. BJPsych Open 7(1):e17, 2020 33308363

Hersh R, Caligor E, Yeomans FE, et al: Fundamentals of TFP: Applications in Psychiatric and General Medical Settings. New York, Springer, 2017

Hilden HM, Rosenström T, Karila I, et al: Effectiveness of brief schema group therapy for borderline personality disorder symptoms: a randomized pilot study. Nord J Psychiatry 75(3):176–185, 2021 33103925

Høgh Egmose C, Heinsvig Poulsen C, Hjorthøj C, et al: The effectiveness of peer support in personal and clinical recovery: systematic review and meta-analysis. Psychiatr Serv 74(8):847–858, 2023 36751908

Hollander E, Allen A, Lopez RP, et al: A preliminary double-blind, placebo-controlled trial of divalproex sodium in borderline personality disorder. J Clin Psychiatry 62(3):199–203, 2001 11305707

Hong V: Borderline personality disorder in the emergency department: good psychiatric management. Harv Rev Psychiatry 24(5):357–366, 2016 27603743

Horvitz-Lennon M, Donohue JM, Domino ME, et al: Improving quality and diffusing best practices: the case of schizophrenia. Health Aff (Millwood) 28(3):701–712, 2009a 19414878

Horvitz-Lennon M, Reynolds S, Wolbert R, et al: The role of assertive community treatment in the treatment of people with borderline personality disorder. Am J Psychiatr Rehabil 12(3):261–277, 2009b 20514357

Howard R, Hasin D, Stohl M: Substance use disorders and criminal justice contact among those with co-occurring antisocial and borderline personality disorders: findings from a nationally representative sample. Personal Ment Health 15(1):40–48, 2021 32588546

Hudays A, Gallagher R, Hazazi A, et al: Eye movement desensitization and reprocessing versus cognitive behavior therapy for treating post-traumatic stress disorder: a systematic review and meta-analysis. Int J Environ Res Public Health 19(24):16836, 2022 36554717

Huo Y, Couzner L, Windsor T, et al: Barriers and enablers for the implementation of trauma-informed care in healthcare settings: a systematic review. Implement Sci Commun 4(1):49, 2023 37147695

Hutsebaut J, Feenstra DJ, Kamphuis JH: Development and preliminary psychometric evaluation of a brief self-report questionnaire for the assessment of the DSM-5 level of Personality Functioning Scale: the LPFS Brief Form (LPFS-BF). Personal Disord 7(2):192–197, 2016 26595344

Ilagan GS, Choi-Kain LW: General psychiatric management for adolescents (GPM-A) with borderline personality disorder. Curr Opin Psychol 37:1–6, 2021 32634737

Iliakis EA, Sonley AKI, Ilagan GS, et al: Treatment of borderline personality disorder: is supply adequate to meet public health needs? Psychiatr Serv 70(9):772–781, 2019 31138059

Iliakis EA, Ilagan GS, Choi-Kain LW: Dropout rates from psychotherapy trials for borderline personality disorder: a meta-analysis. Personal Disord 12(3):193–206, 2021 33591777

Institute for Safe Medication Practice: Implement strategies to prevent persistent medication errors and hazards. Institute for Safe Medication Practices, March 23, 2023. Available at: https://www.ismp.org/resources/implement-strategies-prevent-persistent-medication-errors-and-hazards. Accessed April 4, 2023.

Institute of Medicine: Committee on Quality of Health Care in America: Crossing the Quality Chasm: A New Health System for the 21st Century. Washington, DC, National Academies Press, 2001

Institute of Medicine: Clinical Practice Guidelines We Can Trust. Washington, DC, National Academies Press, 2011

Iyer SP, Spaeth-Rublee B, Pincus HA: Challenges in the operationalization of mental health quality measures: an assessment of alternatives. Psychiatr Serv 67(10):1057–1059, 2016 27301768

Johnson KB, Neuss MJ, Detmer DE: Electronic health records and clinician burnout: a story of three eras. J Am Med Inform Assoc 28(5):967–973, 2021 33367815

Jørgensen CR, Freund C, Bøye R, et al: Outcome of mentalization-based and supportive psychotherapy in patients with borderline personality disorder: a randomized trial. Acta Psychiatr Scand 127(4):305–317, 2013 22897123

Jørgensen MS, Storebø OJ, Stoffers-Winterling JM, et al: Psychological therapies for adolescents with borderline personality disorder (BPD) or BPD features: a systematic review of randomized clinical trials with meta-analysis and trial sequential analysis. PLoS One 16(1):e0245331, 2021 33444397

Jowett S, Karatzias T, Albert I: Multiple and interpersonal trauma are risk factors for both post-traumatic stress disorder and borderline personality disorder: a systematic review on the traumatic backgrounds and clinical characteristics of comorbid post-traumatic stress disorder/borderline personality disorder groups versus single-disorder groups. Psychol Psychother 93(3):621–638, 2020a 31444863

Jowett S, Karatzias T, Shevlin M, et al: Differentiating symptom profiles of ICD-11 PTSD, complex PTSD, and borderline personality disorder: a latent class analysis in a multiply traumatized sample. Personal Disord 11(1):36–45, 2020b 31259603

Juurlink TT, Vukadin M, Stringer B, et al: Barriers and facilitators to employment in borderline personality disorder: a qualitative study among patients, mental health practitioners and insurance physicians. PLoS One 14(7):e0220233, 2019 31335909

Kaba F, Lewis A, Glowa-Kollisch S, et al: Solitary confinement and risk of self-harm among jail inmates. Am J Public Health 104(3):442–447, 2014 24521238

Kadra-Scalzo G, Garland J, Miller S, et al: Comparing psychotropic medication prescribing in personality disorder between general mental health and psychological services: retrospective cohort study. BJPsych Open 7(2):e72, 2021 33762065

Kalira V, Treisman GJ, Clark MR: Borderline personality disorder and chronic pain: a practical approach to evaluation and treatment. Curr Pain Headache Rep 17(8):350, 2013 23801003

Kardas P, Lewek P, Matyjaszczyk M: Determinants of patient adherence: a review of systematic reviews. Front Pharmacol 4:91, 2013 23898295

Kaster TS, Goldbloom DS, Daskalakis ZJ, et al: Electroconvulsive therapy for depression with comorbid borderline personality disorder or post-traumatic stress disorder: a matched retrospective cohort study. Brain Stimul 11(1):204–212, 2018 29111076

Kaufman EA, Xia M, Fosco G, et al: The Difficulties in Emotion Regulation Scale Short Form (DERS-SF): validation and replication in adolescent and adult samples. J Psychopathol Behav Assess 38(3):443–455, 2016

Kay ML, Poggenpoel M, Myburgh CP, et al: Experiences of family members who have a relative diagnosed with borderline personality disorder. Curationis 41(1):e1–e9, 2018 30326706

Kedia SK, Ahuja N, Dillon PJ, et al: Efficacy of extended-release injectable naltrexone on alcohol use disorder treatment: a systematic review. J Psychoactive Drugs 55(2):233–245, 2023 35635191

Kemp K, Zelle H, Bonnie RJ: Embedding advance directives in routine care for persons with serious mental illness: implementation challenges. Psychiatr Serv 66(1):10–14, 2015 25554232

Kessler RC, McGonagle KA, Zhao S, et al: Lifetime and 12-month prevalence of DSM-III-R psychiatric disorders in the United States: results from the National Comorbidity Survey. Arch Gen Psychiatry 51(1):8–19, 1994 8279933

Keuroghlian AS, Gunderson JG, Pagano ME, et al: Interactions of borderline personality disorder and anxiety disorders over 10 years. J Clin Psychiatry 76(11):1529–1534, 2015 26114336

Keuroghlian AS, Palmer BA, Choi-Kain LW, et al: The effect of attending Good Psychiatric Management (GPM) workshops on attitudes toward patients with borderline personality disorder. J Pers Disord 30(4):567–576, 2016 26111249

Kjær JNR, Biskin R, Vestergaard C, et al: All-cause mortality of hospital-treated borderline personality disorder: a nationwide cohort study. J Pers Disord 34(6):723–735, 2020 30307824

Klein P, Fairweather AK, Lawn S: Structural stigma and its impact on healthcare for borderline personality disorder: a scoping review. Int J Ment Health Syst 16(1):48, 2022a 36175958

Klein P, Fairweather AK, Lawn S: The impact of educational interventions on modifying health practitioners' attitudes and practice in treating people with borderline personality disorder: an integrative review. Syst Rev 11(1):108, 2022b 35637499

Kleindienst N, Limberger MF, Ebner-Priemer UW, et al: Dissociation predicts poor response to dialectial behavioral therapy in female patients with borderline personality disorder. J Pers Disord 25(4):432–447, 2011 21838560

Kleindienst N, Jungkunz M, Bohus M: A proposed severity classification of borderline symptoms using the Borderline Symptom List (BSL-23). Borderline Personal Disord Emot Dysregul 7(1):11, 2020 32514359

Klonsky ED, Glenn CR: Assessing the functions of non-suicidal self-injury: psychometric properties of the Inventory of Statements About Self-injury (ISAS). J Psychopathol Behav Assess 31(3):215–219, 2009 29269992

Koivisto M, Melartin T, Lindeman S: Self-invalidation in borderline personality disorder: a content analysis of patients' verbalizations. Psychother Res 32(7):922–935, 2022 35021964

Kolla NJ, Meyer JH, Bagby RM, et al: Trait anger, physical aggression, and violent offending in antisocial and borderline personality disorders. J Forensic Sci 62(1):137–141, 2017 27859182

Konstantinou GN, Trevizol AP, Downar J, et al: Repetitive transcranial magnetic stimulation in patients with borderline personality disorder: a systematic review. Psychiatry Res 304:114145, 2021 34358761

Kramer U, Berger T, Kolly S, et al: Effects of motive-oriented therapeutic relationship in early-phase treatment of borderline personality disorder: a pilot study of a randomized trial. J Nerv Ment Dis 199(4):244–250, 2011 21451348

Kramer U, Kolly S, Berthoud L, et al: Effects of motive-oriented therapeutic relationship in a ten-session general psychiatric treatment of borderline personality disorder: a randomized controlled trial. Psychother Psychosom 83(3):176–186, 2014 24752034

Krause-Utz A: Dissociation, trauma, and borderline personality disorder. Borderline Personal Disord Emot Dysregul 9(1):14, 2022 35440020

Krueger RF, Hobbs KA: An overview of the DSM-5 Alternative Model of Personality Disorders. Psychopathology 53(3–4):126–132, 2020 32645701

Kvarstein EH, Pedersen G, Urnes Ø, et al: Changing from a traditional psychodynamic treatment programme to mentalization-based treatment for patients with borderline personality disorder: does it make a difference? Psychol Psychother 88(1):71–86, 2015 25045028

Lamont E, Dickens GL: Mental health services, care provision, and professional support for people diagnosed with borderline personality disorder: systematic review of service-user, family, and carer perspectives. J Ment Health 30(5):619–633, 2021 31099717

Laporte L, Paris J, Bergevin T, et al: Clinical outcomes of a stepped care program for borderline personality disorder. Personal Ment Health 12(3):252–264, 2018 29709109

Latimer S, Covic T, Tennant A: Co-calibration of deliberate self harm (DSH) behaviours: towards a common measurement metric. Psychiatry Res 200(1):26–34, 2012 22727708

Laurenssen EMP, Luyten P, Kikkert MJ, et al: Day hospital mentalization-based treatment v. specialist treatment as usual in patients with borderline personality disorder: randomized controlled trial. Psychol Med 48(15):2522–2529, 2018 29478425

Le Corff Y, Aluja A, Rossi G, et al: Construct validity of the Dutch, English, French, and Spanish LPFS-BF 2.0: measurement invariance across language and gender and criterion validity. J Pers Disord 36(6):662–679, 2022 36454156

Lee DJ, Witte TK, Bardeen JR, et al: A factor analytic evaluation of the Difficulties in Emotion Regulation Scale. J Clin Psychol 72(9):933–946, 2016 27018649

Lee JH, Kung S, Rasmussen KG, et al: Effectiveness of electroconvulsive therapy in patients with major depressive disorder and comorbid borderline personality disorder. J ECT 35(1):44–47, 2019 30113988

Leichsenring F, Leibing E, Kruse J, et al: Borderline personality disorder. Lancet 377:74–84, 2011 21195251

Leichsenring F, Masuhr O, Jaeger U, et al: Psychoanalytic-interactional therapy versus psychodynamic therapy by experts for personality disorders: a randomized controlled efficacy-effectiveness study in cluster b personality disorders. Psychother Psychosom 85(2):71–80, 2016 26808580

Leichsenring F, Heim N, Leweke F, et al: Borderline personality disorder: a review. JAMA 329(8):670–679, 2023 36853245

Lenzenweger MF, Lane MC, Loranger AW, et al: DSM-IV personality disorders in the National Comorbidity Survey Replication. Biol Psychiatry 62(6):553–564, 2007 17217923

Leppänen V, Hakko H, Sintonen H, et al: Comparing effectiveness of treatments for borderline personality disorder in communal mental health care: The Oulu BPD study. Community Ment Health J 52(2):216–227, 2016 25824852

Lequesne ER, Hersh RG: Disclosure of a diagnosis of borderline personality disorder. J Psychiatr Pract 10(3):170–176, 2004 15330223

Lewis CC, Boyd M, Puspitasari A, et al: Implementing measurement-based care in behavioral health: a review. JAMA Psychiatry 76(3):324–335, 2019 30566197

Lewis-Fernández R, Aggarwal NK, Hinton L, et al (eds): DSM-5 Handbook on the Cultural Formulation Interview. Washington, DC, American Psychiatric Publishing, 2016

Lieslehto J, Tiihonen J, Lähteenvuo M, et al: Comparative effectiveness of pharmacotherapies for the risk of attempted or completed suicide among persons with borderline personality disorder. JAMA Netw Open 6(6):e2317130, 2023 37285156

Lin TJ, Ko HC, Wu JY, et al: The effectiveness of dialectical behavior therapy skills training group vs. cognitive therapy group on reducing depression and suicide attempts for borderline personality disorder in Taiwan. Arch Suicide Res 23(1):82–99, 2019 29528807

Linehan MM: Cognitive-Behavioral Treatment of Borderline Personality Disorder. New York, Guilford, 1993a

Linehan MM1993b: Skills Training Manual for Treating Borderline Personality Disorder. New York, Guilford, 1993b

Linehan MM, Dimeff LA, Reynolds SK, et al: Dialectical behavior therapy versus comprehensive validation therapy plus 12-step for the treatment of opioid dependent women meeting criteria for borderline personality disorder. Drug Alcohol Depend 67(1):13–26, 2002 12062776

Linehan MM, Comtois KA, Murray AM, et al: Two-year randomized controlled trial and follow-up of dialectical behavior therapy vs therapy by experts for suicidal behaviors and borderline personality disorder. Arch Gen Psychiatry 63(7):757–766, 2006 16818865

Linehan MM, McDavid JD, Brown MZ, et al: Olanzapine plus dialectical behavior therapy for women with high irritability who meet criteria for borderline personality disorder: a double-blind, placebo-controlled pilot study. J Clin Psychiatry 69(6):999–1005, 2008 18466045

Linehan MM, Korslund KE, Harned MS, et al: Dialectical behavior therapy for high suicide risk in individuals with borderline personality disorder: a randomized clinical trial and component analysis. JAMA Psychiatry 72(5):475–482, 2015 25806661

Links PL: Handbook of Good Psychiatric Management (GPM) for Borderline Patients. Washington, DC, American Psychiatric Publishing, 2014

Links P, Steiner M, Boiago I, et al: Lithium therapy for borderline patients: preliminary findings. J Pers Disord 4:173–181, 1990

Links PS, Kolla NJ, Guimond T, et al: Prospective risk factors for suicide attempts in a treated sample of patients with borderline personality disorder. Can J Psychiatry 58(2):99–106, 2013 23442897

Links PS, Ross J, Gunderson JG: Promoting good psychiatric management for patients with borderline personality disorder. J Clin Psychol 71(8):753–763, 2015 26197971

Loew TH, Nickel MK, Muehlbacher M, et al: Topiramate treatment for women with borderline personality disorder: a double-blind, placebo-controlled study. J Clin Psychopharmacol 26(1):61–66, 2006 16415708

Lohman MC, Whiteman KL, Yeomans FE, et al: Qualitative analysis of resources and barriers related to treatment of borderline personality disorder in the United States. Psychiatr Serv 68(2):167–172, 2017 27691382

Lyng J, Swales MA, Hastings RP, et al: Standalone DBT group skills training versus standard (i.e., all modes) DBT for borderline personality disorder: a natural quasi-experiment in routine clinical practice. Community Ment Health J 56(2):238–250, 2020 31673877

Machado CDS, Ballester PL, Cao B, et al: Prediction of suicide attempts in a prospective cohort study with a nationally representative sample of the US population. Psychol Med 52(14):2985–2996, 2022 33441206

MacIntyre MR, Appel JM: Legal and ethics considerations in reporting sexual exploitation by previous providers. J Am Acad Psychiatry Law 48(2):166–175, 2020 32051200

MacKinnon R, Michels R, Buckley P: The Psychiatric Interview in Clinical Practice, 3rd Edition. Washington, DC, American Psychiatric Publishing, 2016

Maercker A, Cloitre M, Bachem R, et al: Complex post-traumatic stress disorder. Lancet 400(10345):60–72, 2022 35780794

Maharaj AS, Bhatt NV, Gentile JP: Bringing it in the room: addressing the impact of racism on the therapeutic alliance. Innov Clin Neurosci 18(7–9):39–43, 2021 34980992

Mammen O, Tew J, Painter T, et al: Communicating suicide risk to families of chronically suicidal borderline personality disorder patients to mitigate malpractice risk. Gen Hosp Psychiatry 67:51–57, 2020 33007720

Mannarino VS, Pereira DCS, Gurgel WS, et al: Self-embedding behavior in adults: a report of two cases and a systematic review. J Forensic Sci 62(4):953–961, 2017 27982450

Marino MF, Zanarini MC: Relationship between EDNOS and its subtypes and borderline personality disorder. Int J Eat Disord 29(3):349–353, 2001 11262516

Martin A, Naunton M, Kosari S, et al: Treatment guidelines for PTSD: a systematic review. J Clin Med 10(18):4175, 2021 34575284

Martinussen M, Friborg O, Schmierer P, et al: The comorbidity of personality disorders in eating disorders: a meta-analysis. Eat Weight Disord 22(2):201–209, 2017 27995489

Masland SR, Price D, MacDonald J, et al: Enduring effects of one-day training in good psychiatric management on clinician attitudes about borderline personality disorder. J Nerv Ment Dis 206(11):865–869, 2018 30371640

Masland SR, Victor SE, Peters JR, et al: Destigmatizing borderline personality disorder: a call to action for psychological science. Perspect Psychol Sci 18(2):445–460, 2023 36054911

Masood M: Intentional foreign body ingestions: a complex, recurrent and costly issue. Am J Case Rep 22:e934164, 2021 34780394

Mavranezouli I, Megnin-Viggars O, Daly C, et al: Psychological treatments for post-traumatic stress disorder in adults: a network meta-analysis. Psychol Med 50(4):542–555, 2020 32063234

May T, Pilkington PD, Younan R, et al: Overlap of autism spectrum disorder and borderline personality disorder: a systematic review and meta-analysis. Autism Res 14(12):2688–2710, 2021 34608760

McCauley E, Berk MS, Asarnow JR, et al: Efficacy of dialectical behavior therapy for adolescents at high risk for suicide: a randomized clinical trial. JAMA Psychiatry 75(8):777–785, 2018 29926087

McDermid J, Sareen J, El-Gabalawy R, et al: Co-morbidity of bipolar disorder and borderline personality disorder: findings from the National Epidemiologic Survey on Alcohol and Related Conditions. Compr Psychiatry 58:18–28, 2015 25666748

McGee MD: Cessation of self-mutilation in a patient with borderline personality disorder treated with naltrexone. J Clin Psychiatry 58(1):32–33, 1997 9055839

McGlashan TH, Grilo CM, Skodol AE, et al: The Collaborative Longitudinal Personality Disorders Study: baseline Axis I/II and II/II diagnostic co-occurrence. Acta Psychiatr Scand 102(4):256–264, 2000 11089725

McGonigal PT, Dixon-Gordon KL: Anger and emotion regulation associated with borderline and antisocial personality features within a correctional sample. J Correct Health Care 26(3):215–226, 2020 32787624

McGuinness LA, Higgins JPT: Risk-of-bias VISualization (robvis): an R package and Shiny web app for visualizing risk-of-bias assessments. Res Synth Methods 12(1):55–61, 2021 32336025

McHugh RK, Whitton SW, Peckham AD, et al: Patient preference for psychological vs pharmacologic treatment of psychiatric disorders: a meta-analytic review. J Clin Psychiatry 74(6):595–602, 2013 23842011

McHugo GJ, Krassenbaum S, Donley S, et al: The prevalence of traumatic brain injury among people with co-occurring mental health and substance use disorders. J Head Trauma Rehabil 32(3):E65–E74, 2017 27455436

McIntyre RS, Rosenblat JD, Nemeroff CB, et al: Synthesizing the evidence for ketamine and esketamine in treatment-resistant depression: an international expert opinion on the available evidence and implementation. Am J Psychiatry 178(5):383–399, 2021 33726522

McKenzie K, Gregory J, Hogg L: Mental health workers' attitudes towards individuals with a diagnosis of borderline personality disorder: a systematic literature review. J Pers Disord 36(1):70–98, 2022 34124949

McMain SF, Links PS, Gnam WH, et al: A randomized trial of dialectical behavior therapy versus general psychiatric management for borderline personality disorder. Am J Psychiatry 166(12):1365–1374, 2009 19755574

McMain SF, Guimond T, Streiner DL, et al: Dialectical behavior therapy compared with general psychiatric management for borderline personality disorder: clinical outcomes and functioning over a 2-year follow-up. Am J Psychiatry 169(6):650–661, 2012 22581157

McMain SF, Guimond T, Barnhart R, et al: A randomized trial of brief dialectical behaviour therapy skills training in suicidal patients suffering from borderline disorder. Acta Psychiatr Scand 135(2):138–148, 2017 27858962

Menschner C, Maul A: Key ingredients for successful trauma-informed care implementation. Advancing Trauma-Informed Care, April 2016. Available at: https://www.samhsa.gov/sites/default/files/programs_campaigns/childrens_mental_health/atc-whitepaper-040616.pdf. Accessed August 27, 2023.

Mental Health America: Mental Health America (website). 2023. Available at: https://www.mhanational.org. Accessed May 6, 2023.

Milinkovic MS, Tiliopoulos N: A systematic review of the clinical utility of the DSM-5 section III alternative model of personality disorder. Personal Disord 11(6):377–397, 2020 32324009

Miller AE, Trolio V, Halicki-Asakawa A, et al: Eating disorders and the nine symptoms of borderline personality disorder: a systematic review and series of meta-analyses. Int J Eat Disord 55(8):993–1011, 2022 35579043

Miller CE, Townsend ML, Grenyer BFS: Understanding chronic feelings of emptiness in borderline personality disorder: a qualitative study. Borderline Personal Disord Emot Dysregul 8(1):24, 2021 34365966

Mintz AR, Dobson KS, Romney DM: Insight in schizophrenia: a meta-analysis. Schizophr Res 61(1):75–88, 2003 12648738

Mir J, Kastner S, Priebe S, et al: Treating substance abuse is not enough: comorbidities in consecutively admitted female prisoners. Addict Behav 46:25–30, 2015 25770695

Mirbahaeddin E, Chreim S: A narrative review of factors influencing peer support role implementation in mental health systems: implications for research, policy and practice. Adm Policy Ment Health 49(4):596–612, 2022 35018509

Moen R, Freitag M, Miller M, et al: Efficacy of extended-release divalproex combined with "condensed" dialectical behavior therapy for individuals with borderline personality disorder. Ann Clin Psychiatry 24(4):255–260, 2012 23145381

Mohamed S, Rosenheck R, McEvoy J, et al: Cross-sectional and longitudinal relationships between insight and attitudes toward medication and clinical outcomes in chronic schizophrenia. Schizophr Bull 35(2):336–346, 2009 18586692

Moher D, Shamseer L, Clarke M, et al: Preferred Reporting Items for Systematic Review and Meta-Analysis protocols (PRISMA-P) 2015 statement. Syst Rev 4(1):1, 2015 25554246

Momen NC, Plana-Ripoll O, Yilmaz Z, et al: Comorbidity between eating disorders and psychiatric disorders. Int J Eat Disord 55(4):505–517, 2022 35084057

Morosini PL, Magliano L, Brambilla L, et al: Development, reliability and acceptability of a new version of the DSM-IV Social and Occupational Functioning Assessment Scale (SOFAS) to assess routine social functioning. Acta Psychiatr Scand 101(4):323–329, 2000 10782554

Morton J, Snowdon S, Gopold M, et al: Acceptance and commitment therapy group treatment for symptoms of borderline personality disorder: a public sector pilot study. Cogn Behav Pract 19:527–544, 2012

Moscicki EK, Clarke DE, Kuramoto SJ, et al: Testing DSM-5 in routine clinical practice settings: feasibility and clinical utility. Psychiatr Serv 64(10):952–960, 2013 23852272

Murphy CE 4th, Wang RC, Montoy JC, et al: Effect of extended-release naltrexone on alcohol consumption: a systematic review and meta-analysis. Addiction 117(2):271–281, 2022 34033183

Murray H, Wortzel HS: Psychiatric advance directives: origins, benefits, challenges, and future directions. J Psychiatr Pract 25(4):303–307, 2019 31291211

Nadort M, Arntz A, Smit JH, et al: Implementation of outpatient schema therapy for borderline personality disorder with versus without crisis support by the therapist outside office hours: a randomized trial. Behav Res Ther 47(11):961–973, 2009 19698939

Nakic M, Stefanovics EA, Rhee TG, Rosenheck RA: Lifetime risk and correlates of incarceration in a nationally representative sample of U.S. adults with non-substance-related mental illness. Soc Psychiatry Psychiatr Epidemiol 57(9):1839–1847, 2022 34453553

Narrow WE, Clarke DE, Kuramoto SJ, et al: DSM-5 field trials in the United States and Canada, part III: development and reliability testing of a cross-cutting symptom assessment for DSM-5. Am J Psychiatry 170(1):71–82, 2013 23111499

National Alliance on Mental Illness: NAMI Family and Friends. Arlington, VA, National Alliance on Mental Illness, 2023. Available at: https://www.nami.org/find-support/nami-programs/nami-family-friends. Accessed May 6, 2023.

National Commission on Correctional Health Care: Position statement: solitary confinement (isolation). J Correct Health Care 22(3):257–263, 2016 27302711

National Council for Mental Wellbeing: Fostering Resilience and Recovery: A Change Package. Washington, DC, National Council for Mental Wellbeing, 2019. Available from: https://www.thenationalcouncil.org/resources/fostering-resilience-and-recovery. Accessed August 27, 2023.

National Education Alliance for Borderline Personality Disorder: Books and Publications. Washington, NJ, National Education Alliance for Borderline Personality Disorder, 2023a. Available at: https://www.borderlinepersonalitydisorder.org/books-publications-2. Accessed May 8, 2023.

National Education Alliance for Borderline Personality Disorder: Family Connections Program. Washington, NJ, National Education Alliance for Borderline Personality Disorder, 2023b. Available at: https://www.borderlinepersonalitydisorder.org/family-connections-programs. Accessed May 6, 2023.

National Education Alliance for Borderline Personality Disorder: National Education Alliance for Borderline Personality Disorder (website). Washington, NJ, National Education Alliance for Borderline Personality Disorder, 2023c. Available at: https://www.borderlinepersonalitydisorder.org. Accessed May 6, 2023.

National Health and Medical Research Council: Clinical Practice Guideline for the Management of Borderline Personality Disorder. Melbourne, Australia, National Health and Medical Research Council, 2012. Available at: https://bpdfoundation.org.au/images/mh25_borderline_personality_guideline.pdf. Accessed April 28, 2023.

National Institute for Health and Care Excellence: Borderline Personality Disorder: Recognition and Management. London, National Institute for Health and Care Excellence, 2009. Available at: https://www.nice.org.uk/guidance/cg78/resources/borderline-personality-disorder-recognition-and-management-pdf-975635141317. Accessed April 28, 2023.

National Institute of Mental Health: Borderline personality disorder, in Mental Health Information: Health Topics. Bethesda, MD, National Institute of Mental Health, 2023. Available at: https://www.nimh.nih.gov/health/topics/borderline-personality-disorder. Accessed April 26, 2023.

Navarro-Haro MV, Botella C, Guillen V, et al: Dialectical behavior therapy in the treatment of borderline personality disorder and eating disorders comorbidity: a pilot study in a naturalistic setting. Cognit Ther Res 42:636–649, 2018

Navarro-Haro MV, Botella VG, Badenes-Ribera L, et al: Dialectical behavior therapy in the treatment of co-morbid borderline personality disorder and eating disorder in a naturalistic setting: a six-year follow-up study. Cognit Ther Res 45:480–493, 2021

Neukel C, Bullenkamp R, Moessner M, et al: Anger instability and aggression in borderline personality disorder: an ecological momentary assessment study. Borderline Personal Disord Emot Dysregul 9(1):29, 2022 36244971

Neumann A, van Lier PA, Gratz KL, et al: Multidimensional assessment of emotion regulation difficulties in adolescents using the Difficulties in Emotion Regulation Scale. Assessment 17(1):138–149, 2010 19915198

New York Presbyterian Hospital: Borderline Personality Disorder Resource Center. New York, New York Presbyterian Hospital, 2023. Available at: https://www.nyp.org/bpdresourcecenter. Accessed August 30, 2023.

Ng FY, Bourke ME, Grenyer BF: Recovery from borderline personality disorder: a systematic review of the perspectives of consumers, clinicians, family and carers. PLoS One 11(8):e0160515, 2016 27504634

Ng FYY, Carter PE, Bourke ME, et al: What do individuals with borderline personality disorder want from treatment? A study of self-generated treatment and recovery goals. J Psychiatr Pract 25(2):148–155, 2019a 30849065

Ng FYY, Townsend ML, Miller CE, et al: The lived experience of recovery in borderline personality disorder: a qualitative study. Borderline Personal Disord Emot Dysregul 6:10, 2019b 31143449

Nickel MK, Nickel C, Mitterlehner FO, et al: Topiramate treatment of aggression in female borderline personality disorder patients: a double-blind, placebo-controlled study. J Clin Psychiatry 65(11):1515–1519, 2004 15554765

Nickel MK, Nickel C, Kaplan P, et al: Treatment of aggression with topiramate in male borderline patients: a double-blind, placebo-controlled study. Biol Psychiatry 57(5):495–499, 2005 15737664

Nickel MK, Muehlbacher M, Nickel C, et al: Aripiprazole in the treatment of patients with borderline personality disorder: a double-blind, placebo-controlled study. Am J Psychiatry 163(5):833–838, 2006 16648324

Nickel MK, Loew TH, Pedrosa Gil F: Aripiprazole in treatment of borderline patients, part II: an 18-month follow-up. Psychopharmacology (Berl) 191(4):1023–1026, 2007 17318503

Niemantsverdriet MBA, Slotema CW, Blom JD, et al: Hallucinations in borderline personality disorder: prevalence, characteristics and associations with comorbid symptoms and disorders. Sci Rep 7(1):13920, 2017 29066713

Niesten IJ, Karan E, Frankenburg FR, et al: Description and prediction of the income status of borderline patients over 10 years of prospective follow-up. Personal Ment Health 10(4):285–292, 2016 26864557

Nieuwlaat R, Wilczynski N, Navarro T, et al: Interventions for enhancing medication adherence. Cochrane Database Syst Rev 2014(11):CD000011, 2014 25412402

Nuij C, van Ballegooijen W, de Beurs D, et al: Safety planning-type interventions for suicide prevention: meta-analysis. Br J Psychiatry 219(2):419–426, 2021 35048835

Office for Civil Rights: HIPAA Privacy Rule and Sharing Information Related to Mental Health. Washington, DC, U.S. Department of Health and Human Services. December 19, 2017. Available at: https://www.hhs.gov/sites/default/files/hipaa-privacy-rule-and-sharing-info-related-to-mental-health.pdf. Accessed November 18, 2018.

Office of the National Coordinator for Health Information Technology: 21st Century Cures Act: Interoperability, Information Blocking, and the ONC Health IT Certification Program. Washington, DC, Office of the National Coordinator for Health Information Technology, 2020. Available at: https://www.healthit.gov/cerus/sites/cerus/files/2020–03/ONC_Cures_Act_Final_Rule_.pdf. Accessed February 1, 2023.

Olbert CM, Nagendra A, Buck B: Meta-analysis of Black vs. White racial disparity in schizophrenia diagnosis in the United States: do structured assessments attenuate racial disparities? J Abnorm Psychol 127(1):104–115, 2018 29094963

Oldham JM: Guideline Watch: Practice Guideline for the Treatment of Patients With Borderline Personality Disorder. Washington, DC, American Psychiatric Association, 2005. Available at: https://psychiatryonline.org/pb/assets/raw/sitewide/practice_guidelines/guidelines/bpd-watch-1410457064610.pdf. Accessed November 29, 2022.

Oldham JM: Borderline personality disorder and suicidality. Am J Psychiatry 163(1):20–26, 2006 16390884

Oldham JM: How will clinicians utilize the alternative DSM-5-TR Section III Model for Personality Disorders in their clinical work? Ask the Expert Column. Focus Am Psychiatr Publ 20(4):411–412, 2022a 37200885

Oldham JM: The therapeutic alliance. J Psychiatr Pract 28(5):353, 2022b 36074103

Oldham JM, Morris LB: The New Personality Self-Portrait: Why You Think, Work, Love, and Act the Way You Do. New York, Bantum Books, 1995

Palmier-Claus JE, Ainsworth J, Machin M, et al: The feasibility and validity of ambulatory self-report of psychotic symptoms using a smartphone software application. BMC Psychiatry 12:172, 2012 23075387

Paris J: Why patients with severe personality disorders are overmedicated. J Clin Psychiatry 76(4):e521, 2015 25919846

Paris J: Suicidality in borderline personality disorder. Medicina (Kaunas) 55(6):223, 2019 31142033

Parsons B, Quitkin FM, McGrath PJ, et al: Phenelzine, imipramine, and placebo in borderline patients meeting criteria for atypical depression. Psychopharmacol Bull 25(4):524–534, 1989 2698483

Pascual JC, Soler J, Puigdemont D, et al: Ziprasidone in the treatment of borderline personality disorder: a double-blind, placebo-controlled, randomized study. J Clin Psychiatry 69(4):603–608, 2008 18251623

Pascual JC, Palomares N, Ibáñez Á, et al: Efficacy of cognitive rehabilitation on psychosocial functioning in borderline personality disorder: a randomized controlled trial. BMC Psychiatry 15:255, 2015 26487284

Pascual JC, Arias L, Soler J: Pharmacological management of borderline personality disorder and common comorbidities. CNS Drugs 37(6):489–497, 2023 37256484

Patel MM, Brown JD, Croake S, et al: The current state of behavioral health quality measures: where are the gaps? Psychiatr Serv 66(8):865–871, 2015 26073415

Peh KQE, Kwan YH, Goh H, et al: An adaptable framework for factors contributing to medication adherence: results from a systematic review of 102 conceptual frameworks. J Gen Intern Med 36(9):2784–2795, 2021 33660211

Penner F, Steinberg L, Sharp C: The development and validation of the Difficulties in Emotion Regulation Scale–8: providing respondents with a uniform context that elicits thinking about situations requiring emotion regulation. J Pers Assess 28:1–10, 2022 36306434

Pfohl B, Blum N, St John D, et al: Reliability and validity of the Borderline Evaluation of Severity Over Time (BEST): a self-rated scale to measure severity and change in persons with borderline personality disorder. J Pers Disord 23(3):281–293, 2009 19538082

Philips B, Wennberg P, Konradsson P, et al: Mentalization-based treatment for concurrent borderline personality disorder and substance use disorder: a randomized controlled feasibility study. Eur Addict Res 24(1):1–8, 2018 29402870

Philipsen A, Limberger MF, Lieb K, et al: Attention-deficit hyperactivity disorder as a potentially aggravating factor in borderline personality disorder. Br J Psychiatry 192(2):118–123, 2008 18245028

Pincus HA, Scholle SH, Spaeth-Rublee B, et al: Quality measures for mental health and substance use: gaps, opportunities, and challenges. Health Aff (Millwood) 35(6):1000–1008, 2016 27269015

Porter C, Palmier-Claus J, Branitsky A, et al: Childhood adversity and borderline personality disorder: a meta-analysis. Acta Psychiatr Scand 141(1):6–20, 2020 31630389

Prevolnik Rupel V, Jagger B, Fialho LS, et al: Standard set of patient-reported outcomes for personality disorder. Qual Life Res 30(12):3485–3500, 2021 34075531

Proctor JM, Lawn S, McMahon J: Consumer perspective from people with a diagnosis of borderline personality disorder (BPD) on BPD management-How are the Australian NHMRC BPD guidelines faring in practice? J Psychiatr Ment Health Nurs 28(4):670–681, 2021 33202081

Qadeer Shah A, Prasad D, Caropreso L, et al: The comorbidity between borderline personality disorder (BPD) and generalized anxiety disorder (GAD): a systematic review and meta-analysis. J Psychiatr Res 164:304–314, 2023 37392720

Qian X, Townsend ML, Tan WJ, et al: Sex differences in borderline personality disorder: a scoping review. PLoS One 17(12):e0279015, 2022 36584029

Rada RT, James W: Urethral insertion of foreign bodies: a report of contagious self-mutilation in a maximum-security hospital. Arch Gen Psychiatry 39(4):423–429, 1982 7065851

Raja S, Hasnain M, Hoersch M, et al: Trauma informed care in medicine: current knowledge and future research directions. Fam Community Health 38(3):216–226, 2015 26017000

Rasmussen KG: Do patients with personality disorders respond differentially to electroconvulsive therapy? A review of the literature and consideration of conceptual issues. J ECT 31(1):6–12, 2015 25054362

Reas DL, Rø Ø, Karterud S, et al: Eating disorders in a large clinical sample of men and women with personality disorders. Int J Eat Disord 46(8):801–809, 2013 23983043

Reich DB, Zanarini MC, Bieri KA: A preliminary study of lamotrigine in the treatment of affective instability in borderline personality disorder. Int Clin Psychopharmacol 24(5):270–275, 2009 19636254

Reingle Gonzalez JM, Connell NM: Mental health of prisoners: identifying barriers to mental health treatment and medication continuity. Am J Public Health 104(12):2328–2333, 2014 25322306

Reisner AD, Bornovalova MA, Gordish L, et al: Ingestion of foreign objects as a means of nonlethal self-injury. Personal Disord 4(2):182–189, 2013 22642460

Reneses B, Galián M, Serrano R, et al: A new time limited psychotherapy for BPD: preliminary results of a randomized and controlled trial. Actas Esp Psiquiatr 41(3):139–148, 2013 23803797

Reyes-López J, Ricardo-Garcell J, Armas-Castañeda G, et al: Clinical improvement in patients with borderline personality disorder after treatment with repetitive transcranial magnetic stimulation: preliminary results. Br J Psychiatry 40(1):97–104, 2018 28614492

Rhee TG, Shim SR, Forester BP, et al: Efficacy and safety of ketamine vs electroconvulsive therapy among patients with major depressive episode: a systematic review and meta-analysis. JAMA Psychiatry 79(12):1162–1172, 2022 36260324

Ripoll LH: Psychopharmacologic treatment of borderline personality disorder. Dialogues Clin Neurosci 15(2):213–224, 2013 24174895

Ritschel LA, Tone EB, Schoemann AM, et al: Psychometric properties of the Difficulties in Emotion Regulation Scale across demographic groups. Psychol Assess 27(3):944–954, 2015 25774638

Robinson P, Hellier J, Barrett B, et al: The NOURISHED randomised controlled trial comparing mentalisation-based treatment for eating disorders (MBT-ED) with specialist supportive clinical management (SSCM-ED) for patients with eating disorders and symptoms of borderline personality disorder. Trials 17(1):549, 2016 27855714

Rodriguez-Seijas C, Morgan TA, Zimmerman M: Is there a bias in the diagnosis of borderline personality disorder among lesbian, gay, and bisexual patients? Assessment 28(3):724–738, 2021 32981328

Rodriguez-Seijas C, Rogers BG, Asadi S: Personality disorders research and social decontextualization: what it means to be a minoritized human. Personal Disord 14(1):29–38, 2023 36848071

Rohde C, Polcwiartek C, Correll CU, Nielsen J: Real-world effectiveness of clozapine for borderline personality disorder: results from a 2-year mirror-image study. J Pers Disord 32(6):823–837, 2018 29120277

Romanowicz M, Schak KM, Vande Voort JL, et al: Prescribing practices for patients with borderline personality disorder during psychiatric hospitalizations. J Pers Disord 34(6):736–749, 2020 30742548

Roth AS, Ostroff RB, Hoffman RE: Naltrexone as a treatment for repetitive self-injurious behaviour: an open-label trial. J Clin Psychiatry 57(6):233–237, 1996 8666558

Rudge S, Feigenbaum JD, Fonagy P: Mechanisms of change in dialectical behaviour therapy and cognitive behaviour therapy for borderline personality disorder: a critical review of the literature. J Ment Health 29(1):92–102, 2020 28480806

Rudolph K: Ethical considerations in trauma-informed care. Psychiatr Clin North Am 44(4):521–535, 2021 34763786

Sachdeva S, Goldman G, Mustata G, et al: Naturalistic outcomes of evidence-based therapies for borderline personality disorder at a university clinic: a quasi-randomized trial. J Am Psychoanal Assoc 61(3):578–584, 2013 23720029

Sachs HC, Committee On Drugs: The transfer of drugs and therapeutics into human breast milk: an update on selected topics. Pediatrics 132(3):e796–e809, 2013 23979084

Saks ER: Some thoughts on denial of mental illness. Am J Psychiatry 166(9):972–973, 2009 19723794

Sansone RA, Sansone LA: Measuring self-harm behavior with the self-harm inventory. Psychiatry (Edgmont) 7(4):16–20, 2010 20508804

Sansone RA, Sansone LA: Chronic pain syndromes and borderline personality. Innov Clin Neurosci 9(1):10–14, 2012 22347686

Sansone RA, Levitt JL, Sansone LA: The prevalence of personality disorders among those with eating disorders. Eat Disord 13(1):7–21, 2005 16864328

Santisteban DA, Mena MP, Muir J, et al: The efficacy of two adolescent substance abuse treatments and the impact of comorbid depression: results of a small randomized controlled trial. Psychiatr Rehabil J 38(1):55–64, 2015 25799306

Santo T Jr, Campbell G, Gisev N, et al: Prevalence of mental disorders among people with opioid use disorder: a systematic review and meta-analysis. Drug Alcohol Depend 238:109551, 2022 35797876

Saunders KRK, McGuinness E, Barnett P, et al: A scoping review of trauma informed approaches in acute, crisis, emergency, and residential mental health care. BMC Psychiatry 23(1):567, 2023 37550650

Scalabrini A, Cavicchioli M, Fossati A, et al: The extent of dissociation in borderline personality disorder: a meta-analytic review. J Trauma Dissociation 18(4):522–543, 2017 27681284

Schechter M, Ronningstam E, Herbstman B, et al: Psychotherapy with suicidal patients: the integrative psychodynamic approach of the Boston Suicide Study Group. Medicina (Kaunas) 55(6):303, 2019 31238582

Scheiderer EM, Wood PK, Trull TJ: The comorbidity of borderline personality disorder and posttraumatic stress disorder: revisiting the prevalence and associations in a general population sample. Borderline Personal Disord Emot Dysregul 2:11, 2015 26401313

Schmidt C, Soler J, Carmona I Farrés C, et al: Mindfulness in borderline personality disorder: decentering mediates the effectiveness. Psicothema 33(3):407–414, 2021 34297670

Schneider F, Erhart M, Hewer W, et al: Mortality and medical comorbidity in the severely mentally ill. Dtsch Arztebl Int 116(23–24):405–411, 2019 31366432

Schulz SC, Zanarini MC, Bateman A, et al: Olanzapine for the treatment of borderline personality disorder: variable dose 12-week randomised double-blind placebo-controlled study. Br J Psychiatry 193(6):485–492, 2008 19043153

Schwartz RC, Blankenship DM: Racial disparities in psychotic disorder diagnosis: a review of empirical literature. World J Psychiatry 4(4):133–140, 2014 25540728

Sederer LI, Ellison J, Keyes C: Guidelines for prescribing psychiatrists in consultative, collaborative, and supervisory relationships. Psychiatr Serv 49(9):1197–1202, 1998 9735962

Seid AK, Hesse M, Houborg E, et al: Substance use and violent victimization: evidence from a cohort of >82,000 patients treated for alcohol and drug use disorder in Denmark. J Interpers Violence 37(13–14):NP12427–NP12452, 2022 33719700

Semenza DC, Grosholz JM: Mental and physical health in prison: how co-occurring conditions influence inmate misconduct. Health Justice 7(1):1, 2019 30612284

Shah R, Temes CM, Frankenburg FR, et al: Levels of depersonalization and derealization reported by recovered and non-recovered borderline patients over 20 years of prospective follow-up. J Trauma Dissociation 21(3):337–348, 2020 32000616

Shapiro-Thompson R, Fineberg SK: The state of overmedication in borderline personality disorder: interpersonal and structural factors. Curr Treat Options Psychiatry 9(1):1–13, 2022 36185615

Sharp C: Bridging the gap: the assessment and treatment of adolescent personality disorder in routine clinical care. Arch Dis Child 102(1):103–108, 2017 27507846

Sharp C, Fonagy P: Practitioner review: borderline personality disorder in adolescence: recent conceptualization, intervention, and implications for clinical practice. J Child Psychol Psychiatry 56(12):1266–1288, 2015 26251037

Sharp C, Wall K: Personality pathology grows up: adolescence as a sensitive period. Curr Opin Psychol 21:111–116, 2018 29227834

Sharp C, Wall K: DSM-5 level of personality functioning: refocusing personality disorder on what it means to be human. Annu Rev Clin Psychol 17:313–337, 2021 33306924

Sharp C, Mosko O, Chang B, et al: The cross-informant concordance and concurrent validity of the Borderline Personality Features Scale for Children in a community sample of boys. Clin Child Psychol Psychiatry 16(3):335–349, 2011 20921039

Sharp C, Steinberg L, Temple J, et al: An 11-item measure to assess borderline traits in adolescents: refinement of the BPFSC using IRT. Personal Disord 5(1):70–78, 2014 24588063

Sharp C, Kerr S, Barkauskiene R: The incremental utility of maladaptive self and identity functioning over general functioning for borderline personality disorder features in adolescents. Personal Disord 13(5):474–481, 2022 35201822

Sheehan L, Nieweglowski K, Corrigan P: The stigma of personality disorders. Curr Psychiatry Rep 18(1):11, 2016 26780206

Shields LS, Pathare S, van der Ham AJ, et al: A review of barriers to using psychiatric advance directives in clinical practice. Adm Policy Ment Health 41(6):753–766, 2014 24248818

Silverman MH, Frankenburg FR, Reich DB, et al: The course of anxiety disorders other than PTSD in patients with borderline personality disorder and Axis II comparison subjects: a 10-year follow-up study. J Pers Disord 26(5):804–814, 2012 23013347

Simonsen S, Bateman A, Bohus M, et al: European guidelines for personality disorders: past, present and future. Borderline Personal Disord Emot Dysregul 6:9, 2019 31143448

Simpson EB, Yen S, Costello E, et al: Combined dialectical behavior therapy and fluoxetine in the treatment of borderline personality disorder. J Clin Psychiatry 65(3):379–385, 2004 15096078

Sims E, Nelson KJ, Sisti D: Borderline personality disorder, therapeutic privilege, integrated care: is it ethical to withhold a psychiatric diagnosis? J Med Ethics 48(11):801–804, 2022 34261801

Sinnaeve R, van den Bosch LMC, Hakkaart-van Roijen L, et al: Effectiveness of step-down versus outpatient dialectical behaviour therapy for patients with severe levels of borderline personality disorder: a pragmatic randomized controlled trial. Borderline Personal Disord Emot Dysregul 5:12, 2018 30002832

Sisti D, Segal AG, Siegel AM, et al: Diagnosing, disclosing, and documenting borderline personality disorder: a survey of psychiatrists' practices. J Pers Disord 30(6):848–856, 2016 26623537

Skevington SM, Lotfy M, O'Connell KA, et al: The World Health Organization's WHOQOL-BREF quality of life assessment: psychometric properties and results of the international field trial. A report from the WHOQOL group. Qual Life Res 13(2):299–310, 2004 15085902

Skodol AE, Oldham JM (eds): The American Psychiatric Association Publishing Textbook of Personality Disorders, 3rd Edition. Washington, DC, American Psychiatric Association Publishing, 2021

Skodol AE, Oldham JM, Hyler SE, et al: Comorbidity of DSM-III-R eating disorders and personality disorders. Int J Eat Disord 14(4):403–416, 1993 8293022

Skodol AE, Grilo CM, Keyes KM, et al: Relationship of personality disorders to the course of major depressive disorder in a nationally representative sample. Am J Psychiatry 168(3):257–264, 2011 21245088

Skutch JM, Wang SB, Buqo T, et al: Which brief is best? Clarifying the use of three brief versions of the Difficulties in Emotion Regulation Scale. J Psychopathol Behav Assess 41(3):485–494, 2019 34446987

Sledge W, Plakun EM, Bauer S, et al: Psychotherapy for suicidal patients with borderline personality disorder: an expert consensus review of common factors across five therapies. Borderline Personal Disord Emot Dysregul 1:16, 2014 26401300

Slotema CW, Blom JD, Niemantsverdriet MBA, et al: Auditory verbal hallucinations in borderline personality disorder and the efficacy of antipsychotics: a systematic review. Front Psychiatry 9:347, 2018 30108529

Slotema CW, Wilhelmus B, Arends LR, et al: Psychotherapy for posttraumatic stress disorder in patients with borderline personality disorder: a systematic review and meta-analysis of its efficacy and safety. Eur J Psychotraumatol 11(1):1796188, 2020 33062206

Smith FA, Levenson JL, Stern TA: Psychiatric assessment and consultation, in The American Psychiatric Association Publishing Textbook of Psychosomatic Medicine and Consultation-Liaison Psychiatry, 3rd Edition. Edited by Levenson JL. Washington, DC, American Psychiatric Association Publishing, 2019

Smits ML, Feenstra DJ, Eeren HV, et al: Day hospital versus intensive out-patient mentalisation-based treatment for borderline personality disorder: multicentre randomised clinical trial. Br J Psychiatry 216(2):79–84, 2020 30791963

Smits ML, Feenstra DJ, Bales DL, et al: Day hospital versus intensive outpatient mentalization-based treatment: 3-year follow-up of patients treated for borderline personality disorder in a multicentre randomized clinical trial. Psychol Med 52(3):485–495, 2022 32602830

Söderholm JJ, Socada JL, Rosenström T, et al: Borderline personality disorder with depression confers significant risk of suicidal behavior in mood disorder patients-a comparative study. Front Psychiatry 11:290, 2020 32362847

Soler J, Pascual JC, Campins J, et al: Double-blind, placebo-controlled study of dialectical behavior therapy plus olanzapine for borderline personality disorder. Am J Psychiatry 162(6):1221–1224, 2005 15930077

Soler J, Pascual JC, Tiana T, et al: Dialectical behaviour therapy skills training compared to standard group therapy in borderline personality disorder: a 3-month randomised controlled clinical trial. Behav Res Ther 47(5):353–358, 2009 19246029

Soler J, Casellas-Pujol E, Fernández-Felipe I, et al: "Skills for pills": the dialectical-behavioural therapy skills training reduces polypharmacy in borderline personality disorder. Acta Psychiatr Scand 145(4):332–342, 2022 35088405

Solmi M, Dragioti E, Croatto G, et al: Risk and protective factors for personality disorders: an umbrella review of published meta-analyses of case-control and cohort studies. Front Psychiatry 12:679379, 2021 34552513

Soloff PH: Bridging the gap between remission and recovery in BPD: qualitative versus quantitative perspectives. J Pers Disord 35(1):21–40, 2021 30785863

Sommer JL, Blaney C, Mota N, et al: Dissociation as a transdiagnostic indicator of self-injurious behavior and suicide attempts: a focus on posttraumatic stress disorder and borderline personality disorder. J Trauma Stress 34(6):1149–1158, 2021 34426995

Soulier MF, Maislen A, Beck JC: Status of the psychiatric duty to protect, circa 2006. J Am Acad Psychiatry Law 38(4):457–473, 2010 21156904

Spengler ES, Miller DJ, Spengler PM: Microaggressions: clinical errors with sexual minority clients. Psychotherapy (Chic) 53(3):360–366, 2016 27631867

Spinhoven P, Giesen-Bloo J, van Dyck R, et al: The therapeutic alliance in schema-focused therapy and transference-focused psychotherapy for borderline personality disorder. J Consult Clin Psychol 75(1):104–115, 2007 17295569

Stanley B, Brown GK: Safety planning intervention: a brief intervention to mitigate suicide risk. Cogn Behav Pract 19(2):256–264, 2012

Stanley B, Brown GK, Brenner LA, et al: Comparison of the safety planning intervention with follow-up vs usual care of suicidal patients treated in the emergency department. JAMA Psychiatry 75(9):894–900, 2018 29998307

Stapleton A, Wright N: The experiences of people with borderline personality disorder admitted to acute psychiatric inpatient wards: a meta-synthesis. J Ment Health 28(4):443–457, 2019 28686468

Starcevic V, Janca A: Pharmacotherapy of borderline personality disorder: replacing confusion with prudent pragmatism. Curr Opin Psychiatry 31(1):69–73, 2018 29028643

Steadman HJ, Osher FC, Robbins PC, et al: Prevalence of serious mental illness among jail inmates. Psychiatr Serv 60(6):761–765, 2009 19487344

STEPPS: Systems Training for Emotional Predictability and Problem Solving. Level 1 Publishing, 2022. Available at: https://www.steppsforbpd.com. Accessed March 2, 2023.

Sterne JA, Hernán MA, Reeves BC, et al: ROBINS-I: a tool for assessing risk of bias in non-randomised studies of interventions. BMJ 355:i4919, 2016 27733354

Sterne JAC, Savovic J, Page MJ, et al: RoB 2: a revised tool for assessing risk of bias in randomised trials. BMJ 366:l4898, 2019 31462531

Stiles C, Batchelor R, Gumley A, et al: Experiences of stigma and discrimination in borderline personality disorder: a systematic review and qualitative meta-synthesis. J Pers Disord 37(2):177–194, 2023 37002935

Stoffers-Winterling JM, Storebø OJ, Pereira Ribeiro J, et al: Pharmacological interventions for people with borderline personality disorder. Cochrane Database Syst Rev 11(11):CD012956, 2022 36375174

Stone MH: Borderline patients: 25 to 50 years later: with commentary on outcome factors. Psychodyn Psychiatry 45(2):259–296, 2017 28590208

Storebø OJ, Stoffers-Winterling JM, Völlm BA, et al: Psychological therapies for people with borderline personality disorder. Cochrane Database Syst Rev 5(5):CD012955, 2020 32368793

Strub RL, Black FW: The Mental Status Examination in Neurology. Philadelphia, PA, F.A. Davis Co., 2000

Stubbe DE: The therapeutic alliance: the fundamental element of psychotherapy. Focus Am Psychiatr Publ 16(4):402–403, 2018 31975934

Substance Abuse and Mental Health Services Administration: SAFE-T Pocket Card: Suicide and Five-Step Evaluation and Triage. Rockville, MD, Substance Abuse and Mental Health Services Administration, September 2009. Available at: https://store.samhsa.gov/product/SAFE-T-Pocket-Card-Suicide-Assessment-Five-Step-Evaluation-and-Triage-for-Clinicians/sma09-4432. Accessed April 26, 2023.

Substance Abuse and Mental Health Services Administration: SAMHSA's Working Definition of Recovery: 10 Guiding Principles of Recovery. Rockville, MD, Substance Abuse and Mental Health Services Administration, 2012. Available at: https://store.samhsa.gov/sites/default/files/pep12-recdef.pdf. Accessed August 3, 2019.

Substance Abuse and Mental Health Services Administration: SAMHSA's Concept of Trauma and Guidance for a Trauma-Informed Approach. HHS Publ No (SMA) 14-4884. Rockville, MD, Substance Abuse and Mental Health Services Administration, 2014. Available at: https://ncsacw.acf.hhs.gov/userfiles/files/SAMHSA_Trauma.pdf. Accessed August 27, 2023.

Substance Abuse and Mental Health Services Administration: Peer support workers for those in recovery, in Recovery Support Tools and Resources. Rockville, MD, Substance Abuse and Mental Health Services Administration, 2022. Available at: https://www.samhsa.gov/brss-tacs/recovery-support-tools/peers. Accessed September 2, 2023.

Sue DW, Capodilupo CM, Torino GC, et al: Racial microaggressions in everyday life: implications for clinical practice. Am Psychol 62(4):271–286, 2007 17516773

Sulzer SH, Muenchow E, Potvin A, et al: Improving patient-centered communication of the borderline personality disorder diagnosis. J Ment Health 25(1):5–9, 2016 26360788

Tamburello A, Metzner J, Fergusen E, et al: The American Academy of Psychiatry and the Law practice resource for prescribing in corrections. J Am Acad Psychiatry Law 46(2):242–243, 2018 30026404

Tate AE, Sahlin H, Liu S, et al: Borderline personality disorder: associations with psychiatric disorders, somatic illnesses, trauma, and adverse behaviors. Mol Psychiatry 27(5):2514–2521, 2022 35304564

Temes CM, Frankenburg FR, Fitzmaurice GM, et al: Deaths by suicide and other causes among patients with borderline personality disorder and personality-disordered comparison subjects over 24 years of prospective follow-up. J Clin Psychiatry 80(1):18m12436, 2019

The Joint Commission: National Patient Safety Goals® Effective January 2023 for the Hospital Program. Oakbrook Terrace, IL, The Joint Commission, 2022. Available at: https://www.jointcommission.org/-/media/tjc/documents/standards/national-patient-safety-goals/2023/npsg_chapter_hap_jan2023.pdf. Accessed April 4, 2023.

Timäus C, Meiser M, Wiltfang J, et al: Efficacy of naltrexone in borderline personality disorder, a retrospective analysis in inpatients. Hum Psychopharmacol 36(6):e2800, 2021 34029405

Tomko RL, Trull TJ, Wood PK, et al: Characteristics of borderline personality disorder in a community sample: comorbidity, treatment utilization, and general functioning. J Pers Disord 28(5):734–750, 2014 25248122

Tong P, Bo P, Shi Y, et al: Clinical traits of patients with major depressive disorder with comorbid borderline personality disorder based on propensity score matching. Depress Anxiety 38(1):100–106, 2021 33326658

Torgersen J: Textbook of Personality Disorders. Washington, DC, American Psychiatric Publishing, 2005

Tosato S, Albert U, Tomassi S, et al: A systematized review of atypical antipsychotics in pregnant women: balancing between risks of untreated illness and risks of drug-related adverse effects. J Clin Psychiatry 78(5):e477–e489, 2017 28297592

Tritt K, Nickel C, Lahmann C, et al: Lamotrigine treatment of aggression in female borderline-patients: a randomized, double-blind, placebo-controlled study. J Psychopharmacol 19(3):287–291, 2005 15888514

Trull TJ, Jahng S, Tomko RL, et al: Revised NESARC personality disorder diagnoses: gender, prevalence, and comorbidity with substance dependence disorders. J Pers Disord 24(4):412–426, 2010 20695803

Trull TJ, Freeman LK, Vebares TJ, et al: Borderline personality disorder and substance use disorders: an updated review. Borderline Personal Disord Emot Dysregul 5:15, 2018 30250740

Tyrer P, Tom B, Byford S, et al: Differential effects of manual assisted cognitive behavior therapy in the treatment of recurrent deliberate self-harm and personality disturbance: the POPMACT study. J Pers Disord 18(1):102–116, 2004 15061347

U.S. Food and Drug Administration: Drug safety communication: antipsychotic drug labels updated on use during pregnancy and risk of abnormal muscle movements and withdrawal symptoms in newborns. U.S. Food and Drug Administration, February 22, 2011. Available at: https://www.fda.gov/Drugs/DrugSafety/ucm243903.htm#sa. Accessed September 22, 2019.

Üstün TB, Kostanjsek N, Chatterji S, et al: Measuring Health and Disability: Manual for the WHO Disability Assessment Schedule (WHODAS 2.0). Geneva, World Health Organization, 2010

Valenstein M, Adler DA, Berlant J, et al: Implementing standardized assessments in clinical care: now's the time. Psychiatr Serv 60(10):1372–1375, 2009 19797378

van den Bosch LM, Koeter MW, Stijnen T, et al: Sustained efficacy of dialectical behaviour therapy for borderline personality disorder. Behav Res Ther 43(9):1231–1241, 2005 16005708

Van den Eynde V, Abdelmoemin WR, Abraham MM, et al: The prescriber's guide to classic MAO inhibitors (phenelzine, tranylcypromine, isocarboxazid) for treatment-resistant depression. CNS Spectr 15:1–14, 2022a 35837681

Van den Eynde V, Gillman PK, Blackwell BB: The prescriber's guide to the MAOI diet: thinking through tyramine troubles. Psychopharmacol Bull 52(2):73–116, 2022b 35721816

Vanek J, Prasko J, Ociskova M, et al: Insomnia in patients with borderline personality disorder. Nat Sci Sleep 13:239–250, 2021 33654445

Vanicek T, Unterholzner J, Lanzenberger R, et al: Intravenous esketamine leads to an increase in impulsive and suicidal behaviour in a patient with recurrent major depression and borderline personality disorder. World J Biol Psychiatry 23(9):715–718, 2022 35057708

Vanwoerden S, Garey L, Ferguson T, et al: Borderline Personality Features Scale for Children-11: measurement invariance over time and across gender in a community sample of adolescents. Psychol Assess 31(1):114–119, 2019 30080065

Verheul R, Van Den Bosch LM, Koeter MW, et al: Dialectical behaviour therapy for women with borderline personality disorder: 12-month, randomised clinical trial in The Netherlands. Br J Psychiatry 182:135–140, 2003 12562741

Victor G, Hedden-Clayton B: Substance use and violence victimization among women: a review of relevant literature. Violence Vict 38(1):25–52, 2023 36717198

Victor SE, Klonsky ED: Validation of a brief version of the Difficulties in Emotion Regulation Scale (DERS-18) in five samples. J Psychopathol Behav Assess 38(4):582–589, 2016

Videler AC, Hutsebaut J, Schulkens JEM, et al: A life span perspective on borderline personality disorder. Curr Psychiatry Rep 21(7):51, 2019 31161404

Volkert J, Gablonski TC, Rabung S: Prevalence of personality disorders in the general adult population in Western countries: systematic review and meta-analysis. Br J Psychiatry 213(6):709–715, 2018 30261937

Wall K, Ahmed Y, Sharp C: Parent-adolescent concordance in borderline pathology and why it matters. J Abnorm Child Psychol 47(3):529–542, 2019 30062612

Walton CJ, Bendit N, Baker AL, et al: A randomised trial of dialectical behaviour therapy and the conversational model for the treatment of borderline personality disorder with recent suicidal and/or non-suicidal self-injury: an effectiveness study in an Australian public mental health service. Aust N Z J Psychiatry 54(10):1020–1034, 2020 32551819

Wang K, Varma DS, Prosperi M: A systematic review of the effectiveness of mobile apps for monitoring and management of mental health symptoms or disorders. J Psychiatr Res 107:73–78, 2018 30347316

Ward HB, Yip A, Siddiqui R, et al: Borderline personality traits do not influence response to TMS. J Affect Disord 281:834–838, 2021 33229022

Watkins K, Horvitz-Lennon M, Caldarone LB, et al: Developing medical record-based performance indicators to measure the quality of mental healthcare. J Healthc Qual 33(1):49–66, quiz 66–67, 2011 21199073

Watkins KE, Farmer CM, De Vries D, et al: The Affordable Care Act: an opportunity for improving care for substance use disorders? Psychiatr Serv 66(3):310–312, 2015 25727120

Watkins KE, Smith B, Akincigil A, et al: The quality of medication treatment for mental disorders in the Department of Veterans Affairs and in private-sector plans. Psychiatr Serv 67(4):391–396, 2016 26567931

Way BB, Miraglia R, Sawyer DA, et al: Factors related to suicide in New York state prisons. Int J Law Psychiatry 28(3):207–221, 2005 15950281

Weekers LC, Hutsebaut J, Kamphuis JH: The Level of Personality Functioning Scale–Brief Form 2.0: update of a brief instrument for assessing level of personality functioning. Personal Ment Health 13(1):3–14, 2019 30230242

Weinberg I, Gunderson JG, Hennen J, Cutter CJ Jr: Manual assisted cognitive treatment for deliberate self-harm in borderline personality disorder patients. J Pers Disord 20(5):482–492, 2006 17032160

Weiner AS, Ensink K, Normandin L: Psychotherapy for borderline personality disorder in adolescents. Psychiatr Clin North Am 41(4):729–746, 2018 30447735

Wenzlow AT, Ireys HT, Mann B, et al: Effects of a discharge planning program on Medicaid coverage of state prisoners with serious mental illness. Psychiatr Serv 62(1):73–78, 2011 21209303

Wetterborg D, Långström N, Andersson G, et al: Borderline personality disorder: prevalence and psychiatric comorbidity among male offenders on probation in Sweden. Compr Psychiatry 62:63–70, 2015 26343468

WHOQOL Group: Development of the World Health Organization WHOQOL-BREF quality of life assessment. Psychol Med 28(3):551–558, 1998 9626712

Wilder CM, Elbogen EB, Moser LL, et al: Medication preferences and adherence among individuals with severe mental illness and psychiatric advance directives. Psychiatr Serv 61(4):380–385, 2010 20360277

Wilhelmus B, Marissen MAE, van den Berg D, et al: Adding EMDR for PTSD at the onset of treatment of borderline personality disorder: a pilot study. J Behav Ther Exp Psychiatry 79:101834, 2023 36645926

Wilkinson ST, Trujillo Diaz D, Rupp ZW, et al: Pharmacological and somatic treatment effects on suicide in adults: a systematic review and meta-analysis. Focus Am Psychiatr Publ 21(2):197–208, 2023 37201149

Williamson D, Turkoz I, Wajs E, et al: Adverse events and measurement of dissociation after the first dose of esketamine in patients with TRD. Int J Neuropsychopharmacol 26(3):198–206, 2023 36525338

Wilper AP, Woolhandler S, Boyd JW, et al: The health and health care of US prisoners: results of a nationwide survey. Am J Public Health 99(4):666–672, 2009 19150898

Winsper C: Borderline personality disorder: course and outcomes across the lifespan. Curr Opin Psychol 37:94–97, 2021 33091693

Winsper C, Tang NK, Marwaha S, et al: The sleep phenotype of borderline personality disorder: a systematic review and meta-analysis. Neurosci Biobehav Rev 73:48–67, 2017 27988314

Winsper C, Bilgin A, Thompson A, et al: The prevalence of personality disorders in the community: a global systematic review and meta-analysis. Br J Psychiatry 216(2):69–78, 2020 31298170

Woodbridge J, Townsend M, Reis S, et al: Non-response to psychotherapy for borderline personality disorder: a systematic review. Aust N Z J Psychiatry 56(7):771–787, 2022 34525867

Woodbridge J, Townsend ML, Reis SL, et al: Patient perspectives on non-response to psychotherapy for borderline personality disorder: a qualitative study. Borderline Personal Disord Emot Dysregul 10(1):13, 2023 37072881

World Health Organization: International Statistical Classification of Diseases and Related Health Problems, 10th Revision. Geneva, World Health Organization, 1992

Wortzel HS, Simonetti JA, Oslin DW, et al: Lithium use for suicide prevention, revisited. J Psychiatr Pract 29(1):51–57, 2023 36649553

Yadav D: Prescribing in borderline personality disorder: the clinical guidelines. Prog Neurol Psychiatry 24(2):25–30, 2020

Yasmeen S, Tangney JP, Stuewig JB, et al: The implications of borderline personality features for jail inmates' institutional misconduct and treatment-seeking. Personal Disord 13(5):505–515, 2022 34780233

Yen S, Peters JR, Nishar S, et al: Association of borderline personality disorder criteria with suicide attempts: findings from the collaborative longitudinal study of personality disorders over 10 years of follow-up. JAMA Psychiatry 78(2):187–194, 2021 33206138

Yeomans FE, Clarkin JF, Kernberg OF: Transference-Focused Psychotherapy for BPD: A Clinical Guide. Washington, DC, American Psychiatric Publishing, 2015

Yildiz A, Siafis S, Mavridis D, et al: Comparative efficacy and tolerability of pharmacological interventions for acute bipolar depression in adults: a systematic review and network meta-analysis. Lancet Psychiatry 10(9):693–705, 2023 37595997

Young JE, Klosko J, Weishaar ME: Schema Therapy: A Practitioner's Guide. New York, Guilford, 2003

Young MH, Justice JV, Erdberg P: Risk of harm: inmates who harm themselves while in prison psychiatric treatment. J Forensic Sci 51(1):156–162, 2006 16423243

Zanarini MC, Frankenburg FR: Olanzapine treatment of female borderline personality disorder patients: a double-blind, placebo-controlled pilot study. J Clin Psychiatry 62(11):849–854, 2001 11775043

Zanarini MC, Frankenburg FR: A preliminary, randomized trial of psychoeducation for women with borderline personality disorder. J Pers Disord 22(3):284–290, 2008 18540800

Zanarini MC, Gunderson JG, Frankenburg FR, et al: Discriminating borderline personality disorder from other axis II disorders. Am J Psychiatry 147(2):161–167, 1990 2301653

Zanarini MC, Frankenburg FR, Dubo ED, et al: Axis I comorbidity of borderline personality disorder. Am J Psychiatry 155(12):1733–1739, 1998 9842784

Zanarini MC, Vujanovic AA, Parachini EA, et al: Zanarini Rating Scale for Borderline Personality Disorder (ZAN-BPD): a continuous measure of DSM-IV borderline psychopathology. J Pers Disord 17(3):233–242, 2003 12839102

Zanarini MC, Frankenburg FR, Hennen J, et al: Axis I comorbidity in patients with borderline personality disorder: 6-year follow-up and prediction of time to remission. Am J Psychiatry 161(11):2108–2114, 2004a 15514413

Zanarini MC, Frankenburg FR, Hennen J, et al: Mental health service utilization by borderline personality disorder patients and Axis II comparison subjects followed prospectively for 6 years. J Clin Psychiatry 65(1):28–36, 2004b 14744165

Zanarini MC, Frankenburg FR, Parachini EA: A preliminary, randomized trial of fluoxetine, olanzapine, and the olanzapine-fluoxetine combination in women with borderline personality disorder. J Clin Psychiatry 65(7):903–907, 2004c 15291677

Zanarini MC, Frankenburg FR, Reich DB, et al: The 10-year course of physically self-destructive acts reported by borderline patients and Axis II comparison subjects. Acta Psychiatr Scand 117(3):177–184, 2008 18241308

Zanarini MC, Reichman CA, Frankenburg FR, et al: The course of eating disorders in patients with borderline personality disorder: a 10-year follow-up study. Int J Eat Disord 43(3):226–232, 2010 19343799

Zanarini MC, Horwood J, Wolke D, et al: Prevalence of DSM-IV borderline personality disorder in two community samples: 6,330 English 11-year-olds and 34,653 American adults. J Pers Disord 25(5):607–619, 2011a 22023298

Zanarini MC, Schulz SC, Detke HC, et al: A dose comparison of olanzapine for the treatment of borderline personality disorder: a 12-week randomized, double-blind, placebo-controlled study. J Clin Psychiatry 72(10):1353–1362, 2011b 21535995

Zanarini MC, Frankenburg FR, Reich DB, et al: Attainment and stability of sustained symptomatic remission and recovery among patients with borderline personality disorder and Axis II comparison subjects: a 16-year prospective follow-up study. Am J Psychiatry 169(5):476–483, 2012 22737693

Zanarini MC, Weingeroff JL, Frankenburg FR, et al: Development of the self-report version of the Zanarini Rating Scale for Borderline Personality Disorder. Personal Ment Health 9(4):243–249, 2015 26174588

Zanarini MC, Temes CM, Ivey AM, et al: The 10-year course of adult aggression toward others in patients with borderline personality disorder and axis II comparison subjects. Psychiatry Res 252:134–138, 2017 28264784

Zanarini MC, Conkey LC, Temes CM, et al: Randomized controlled trial of web-based psychoeducation for women with borderline personality disorder. J Clin Psychiatry 79(3):79, 2018 28703950

Zanarini MC, Hörz-Sagstetter S, Temes CM, et al: The 24-year course of major depression in patients with borderline personality disorder and personality-disordered comparison subjects. J Affect Disord 258:109–114, 2019 31400625

Zanarini MC, Athanasiadi A, Temes CM, et al: Symptomatic disorders in adults and adolescents with borderline personality disorder. J Pers Disord 35(Suppl B):48–55, 2021 33779275

Zeifman RJ, Landy MSH, Liebman RE, et al: Optimizing treatment for comorbid borderline personality disorder and posttraumatic stress disorder: a systematic review of psychotherapeutic approaches and treatment efficacy. Clin Psychol Rev 86:102030, 2021 33894491

Zimmerman M, Becker L: The hidden borderline patient: patients with borderline personality disorder who do not engage in recurrent suicidal or self-injurious behavior. Psychol Med 53(11):5177–5184, 2023 35903008

Zimmerman M, Mattia JI: Axis I diagnostic comorbidity and borderline personality disorder. Compr Psychiatry 40(4):245–252, 1999 10428182

Zimmermann J, Kerber A, Rek K, et al: A brief but comprehensive review of research on the Alternative DSM-5 Model for Personality Disorders. Curr Psychiatry Rep 21(9):92, 2019 31410586

Zimmerman M, Chelminski I, Young D, et al: Using outcome measures to promote better outcomes. Clin Neuropsychiatry 8:28–36, 2011

Zimmerman M, Chelminski I, Dalrymple K, et al: Principal diagnoses in psychiatric outpatients with borderline personality disorder: implications for screening recommendations. Ann Clin Psychiatry 29(1):54–60, 2017 28207916

Zimmerman M, McGonigal P, Moon SS, et al: Does diagnosing a patient with borderline personality disorder negatively impact patient satisfaction with the initial diagnostic evaluation? Ann Clin Psychiatry 30(3):215–219, 2018 30028896

Zimmerman M, Benjamin I, Seijas-Rodriguez C: Psychiatric diagnoses among transgender and gender diverse patients compared to cisgender patients. J Clin Psychiatry 83(6):21m14062, 2022 36170202

Disclosures

The GWG and SRG reported the following disclosures during development and approval of this guideline:

Dr. Keepers is employed as Professor and Chair of the Department of Psychiatry by Oregon Health & Science University. He receives travel funds from the American Board of Psychiatry and Neurology, the American College of Psychiatry, and the Accreditation Council for Graduate Medical Education related to his activities as a member or chair of various committees. He reports no conflicts of interest with his work on this guideline.

Dr. Fochtmann is employed as a SUNY Distinguished Service Professor of Psychiatry, Pharmacological Sciences, and Biomedical Informatics at Stony Brook University and Deputy Chief Medical Information Officer for Stony Brook Medicine. She also consults for the American Psychiatric Association on the development of practice guidelines. She reports no conflicts of interest with her work on this guideline.

Dr. Anzia is employed as Professor of Psychiatry and Behavioral Sciences and Residency Program Director/Vice Chair for Education at Northwestern University/Feinberg School of Medicine. She receives part of her salary from the Medical Staff Office of Northwestern Medicine for her role as Physician Health Liaison. Dr. Anzia receives travel funds from the American Board of Psychiatry and Neurology, the American College of Psychiatry, and the Accreditation Council for Graduate Medical Education for her activities as Board Director, committee chair, and various other committees. She has no conflicts of interest with her work on this guideline.

Dr. Benjamin is employed as Vice Chair for Education in Psychiatry at the University of Massachusetts T. H. Chan School of Medicine, where he is also Director of Neuropsychiatry and Professor of Psychiatry and Neurology. He periodically receives honoraria for lectures, provides consultation to the Massachusetts Department of Mental Health, and serves as an expert witness on neuropsychiatric issues. He is a partner in and author for Brain Educators, LLC, a publisher of educational materials designed to improve neuropsychiatric assessment skills. Any income received is used to offset production and development costs of the materials. He is a psychiatry director of the American Board of Psychiatry and Neurology and receives a stipend in connection with this work. He reports no conflicts of interest with his work on this guideline.

Dr. Lyness is employed as President and Chief Executive Officer of the American Board of Psychiatry and Neurology. He has an unpaid position as Professor Emeritus of Psychiatry at the University of Rochester School of Medicine & Dentistry. Previously, he was employed as Senior Associate Dean for Academic Affairs and Professor of Psychiatry and Neurology in the School of Medicine & Dentistry at the University of Rochester Medical Center, received compensation as a Psychiatry Director of the American Board of Psychiatry and Neurology, and provided independent medical examinations for various attorneys. He is a paid contributor to several articles for UpToDate, Inc. He has no other relevant financial or fiduciary interests and reports no conflicts of interest with his work on this guideline.

Dr. Mojtabai is employed as Professor of Public Health at Johns Hopkins Bloomberg School of Public Health with joint appointment in the Department of Psychiatry and Behavioral Sciences in Baltimore, Maryland, and as a psychiatrist at Johns Hopkins Hospital. He has been a principal investigator and co-investigator on grants funded by the National Institutes of Health. During the period of working on this guideline, he received royalties from UpToDate, Inc., and provided research consultation to Surgo Ventures as well as expert consultation regarding social media litigation on behalf of the plaintiffs. He reports no conflicts of interest with his work on this guideline.

Dr. Servis is employed as Professor of Psychiatry and Behavioral Sciences and the Vice Dean for Medical Education at the University of California Davis School of Medicine. He consults to the Medical Board of California and serves on the Psychiatry Residency in Training Examination Editorial Board for the American College of Psychiatrists and the Interdisciplinary Review Committee for the USMLE Step 2 Examination for the National Board of Medical Examiners. He reports no conflicts of interest with his work on this guideline.

Dr. Choi-Kain is employed as the Director of the Gunderson Personality Disorders Institute at McLean Hospital as well as an Assistant Professor of Psychiatry at Harvard Medical School. The Gunderson Personality Disorders Institute has a training division, providing formal training in evidence-based treatments, consultations to teams, training of trainers, and supervision of clinicians using these treatments. Dr. Choi-Kain receives payments via McLean Hospital from government agencies in Canada, Australia, Sweden, and others for teaching. The other part of the institute is a research laboratory through which Dr. Choi-Kain receives funding from private funds as well as the National Alliance for Research on Schizophrenia & Depression/Brain & Behavior Research Foundation. She receives royalties from the sales of books on BPD, especially GPM books from Springer and American Psychiatric Association Publishing. Her conflicts of interest with her work on this guideline include her work with GPM, which has been informed by prior guidelines and will incorporate any changed guidelines.

Dr. Nelson is employed as Associate Professor of Psychiatry and Behavioral Sciences and Associate Designated Institutional Official at the University of Minnesota Medical School. Dr. Nelson receives educational research grant support and travel funds from the American Board of Psychiatry and Neurology. Other sources of financial income include honoraria from universities and health systems for providing grand rounds presentations on the topic of BPD and other topics. Dr. Nelson has been compensated for providing consultative services in psychiatric education leadership and administration. Dr. Nelson receives royalties from UpToDate, Inc., and from Oxford University Press. Dr. Nelson receives royalties from Oxford University Press for co-editing a book on the topic of schizophrenia. Dr. Nelson has not received financial support from the pharmaceutical or medical device industry and reports no conflicts of interest with her work on this guideline.

Dr. Sharp is the John and Rebecca Moores Professor and Associate Dean for Faculty and Research in the Psychology Department and clinical program at the University of Houston. She is also the director of the Developmental Psychopathology Lab and the Adolescent Diagnosis Assessment Prevention and Treatment (ADAPT) Center at the University of Houston. Dr. Sharp received funding from the National Institute of Mental Health and National Institute of Child Health and Human Development for several grants on which she is the principal investigator (1R01MH127060-02, 1R01HD102436-01A1, R21MH128570), co-investigator (1R01 MH129354-01, 1I01 CX002135-01A1), faculty sponsor (1F31HD108859-01A1, 1F31MH123127-01A1), or consultant (R21 MH125052-01A1). She received honoraria for providing grand rounds and other types of educational activities related to her expertise in the developmental aspect of personality pathology. She receives royalties from Springer, American Psychiatric Association, Routledge, MIT Press, and Guilford for books on the topic of personality pathology and related pathology and/or caregiving. She is editor of *Personality and Mental Health*, associate editor of *Personality Disorders: Theory, Research and Treatment*, and section editor for *Borderline Personality Disorder and Emotion Dysregulation*.

Dr. Degenhardt is a child and adolescent psychiatrist employed by the Fraser Health Authority specializing in emergency psychiatry and early psychosis. She is also a clinical instructor at the University of British Columbia. During the period of preparation of this guideline, she was employed by Vancouver Coastal Health as she completed her child and adolescent subspecialty training. She reports no conflicts of interest with her work on this guideline.

Dr. Oldham is a Distinguished Emeritus Professor at Baylor College of Medicine and a senior consultant at The Menninger Clinic. He serves as editor for the *Journal of Psychiatric Practice*, co-editor for the *Journal of Personality Disorders*, and joint Editor-in-Chief for *Borderline Personality Disorder and Emotion Dysregulation*. He is an officer of NPSP25, LLC, and a member of the Academic Advisory Board for Silver Hill Hospital. He reports no conflicts of interest with his work on this guideline.

Individuals and Organizations That Submitted Comments

Hira Aslam, M.S., B.S.
Bo Bach, Ph.D.
Lee Anna Clark, Ph.D.
John F. Clarkin, Ph.D.
Katie Dixon-Gordon, Ph.D.
Sarah Fineberg, M.D., Ph.D.
Marianne Goodman, M.D.
Paige Hector, L.M.S.W.
Nathaniel Herr, Ph.D.
Kimberly Hickey, B.A.
Gabrielle Ilagan, M.A.
Lisa Johnson, Ph.D.
Anne Justus, Ph.D.
Harold W. Koenigsberg, M.D.
Paul S. Links, M.D., M.Sc, FRCPC
Rebecca Mardis, B.S.
Shelley McMain, Ph.D., C.Psych.
H. George Nurnberg, M.D., DLFAPA
Desmond Oathes, Ph.D.
Jillian Papa, M.P.H.
Joel Paris, M.D.
K. Hogan Pesaniello, M.D.
Alexandra Philipsen, M.D.
Seth Pitman, Ph.D.

Eric M. Plakun, M.D.
Daniel Roberts, M.D., M.S.W.
Craig Rodriguez-Seijas, Ph.D.
Elsa Ronningstam, Ph.D.
Shira Rubinstein, M.D.
Anthony Ruocco, Ph.D.
Philip S. Santangelo, Ph.D.
Shannon Sauer-Zavala, Ph.D.
Lori Scott, Ph.D.
John Shemo, M.D.
Jonathan Shepherd, M.D.
Laika Simeon-Thompson, M.D.
Andrew Skodol, M.D.
Alexandra G. Stein, B.A.
Saundra Stock, M.D.
Paula Tusiani-Eng, M.Div. L.M.S.W.
Grace Nayla, MRCPsych, ABPsych
Kellyann May Navarre, B.A.
Paula Jimena Zavala Billingsley
　　Zaremba, M.H.S.
Shirley Yen, Ph.D.
Frank Yeomans, M.D.
Mary Zanarini, Ed.D.
Mark Zimmerman, M.D.

AMDA – The Society for Post-Acute and Long-Term Care Medicine
American Academy of Physician Associates
American Association of Geriatric Psychiatry
American College of Neuropsychopharmacology
American Psychiatric Association Council on Research
American Psychological Association
American Society for Adolescent Psychiatry
Association for Behavioral and Cognitive Therapies
Canadian Psychiatric Association
Clinical TMS Society Clinical Standards Committee
DSM Personality Disorder Work Group
Emotions Matter
European Society for the Study of Personality Disorders
International Society for the Study of Personality Disorders
Maryland Psychiatric Society
National Association of State Mental Health Program Directors
National Council for Mental Wellbeing
North American Society for the Study of Personality Disorders
Royal Australian and New Zealand College of Psychiatrists